Understanding and Preventing Student Attrition in Pre-registration Nursing Education

Understanding and Preventing Student Attrition in Pre-registration Nursing Education

DR AMANDA COSTELLO, EdD, MSc, BSc Sociology, PGCE History, NPQH, NPQEL, RNLD
University of Greater Manchester
UK

ELSEVIER

For accessibility purposes, images in electronic versions of this book are accompanied by alt text descriptions provided by Elsevier. For more information, see https://www.elsevier.com/about/accessibility.

Books and journals published by Elsevier comply with applicable product safety requirements. For any product safety concerns or queries, please contact our authorised representative, Elsevier B.V., at productsafety@elsevier.com.

Publisher's note: *Elsevier* takes a neutral position with respect to territorial disputes or jurisdictional claims in its published content, including in maps and institutional affiliations.

Notice

Practitioners and researchers must always rely on their own experience and knowledge in evaluating and using any information, methods, compounds, or experiments described herein. Because of rapid advances in the medical sciences, in particular, independent verification of diagnoses and drug dosages should be made. To the fullest extent of the law, no responsibility is assumed by Elsevier, authors, editors, or contributors for any injury and/or damage to persons or property as a matter of products liability, negligence or otherwise, or from any use or operation of any methods, products, instructions, or ideas contained in the material herein.

ISBN: 978-0-443-40956-1

Executive Content Strategist: Robert Edwards
Content Project Manager: Supriya Barua
Design: Miles Hitchen
Marketing Manager: Deborah J. Watkins

Printed in Great Britain by CPI Group (UK) Ltd,
Croydon CR0 4YY

Last digit is the print number: 9 8 7 6 5 4 3 2 1

PREFACE

Why Are Student Nurses at Risk of Attrition?

Nursing sits at the heart of every healthcare system, yet the journey to becoming a qualified nurse is often far more complex, demanding, and vulnerable to disruption than many outside the profession realise. Around the world, programmes preparing the next generation of nurses face significant challenges, with student attrition emerging as one of the most persistent and costly concerns. This book seeks to highlight why so many aspiring nurses exit their programmes before qualification and, importantly, what can be done to support them to succeed.

The chapters that follow explore this issue from multiple perspectives, beginning with a **historical overview** of nurse education to show how structural shifts, policy reforms, and societal expectations have shaped the student experience. We then provide a clear and research-informed explanation of **what attrition means in the context of higher education,** laying the foundations for understanding the scale and complexity of the problem.

A sample chapter presents **key findings from attrition research conducted in North West England**, offering insight into regional trends that reflect wider national and international patterns. This naturally leads into a detailed examination of the **major factors contributing to attrition** from academic pressures and psychosocial stressors to workplace realities, financial strain, and cultural or gender-related barriers.

Recognising that attrition is never simply statistical, the book also delves into **personal and idiosyncratic reasons for leaving the course,** featuring narratives, case studies, and reflections that reveal the human stories behind the data. The **consequences of attrition**, both for individuals and for healthcare systems, are then explored, highlighting the economic, organisational, and social implications of failing to retain student nurses.

Crucially, this book is not merely diagnostic; it is constructive. A full chapter is devoted to **practical strategies** for reducing attrition, including curriculum redesign, targeted academic support, well-being and mentoring initiatives, improvements to practice placements, and policy shifts at institutional and governmental levels. Examples of **best practice, relevant resources,** and **links to key national and international bodies** round out the text, providing readers with tools for action.

Whether you are an educator, researcher, policymaker, or student, this book aims to equip you with a deeper understanding of attrition's roots and remedies. Above all, it advocates for an educational environment where aspiring nurses are supported, valued, and empowered to fulfil their potential, as the future of healthcare depends on them.

CONTENTS

CHAPTER 1

Historical Context of Nurse Attrition

Amanda Costello

Introduction

The historical context of nursing attrition is the loss of nurses from the workforce, a phenomenon that has long been shaped by the dynamics of the healthcare sector. Attrition is not a new issue; it has roots that stretch back to the earliest days of organised nursing, when the profession began to take form as a vital pillar of public health. Throughout history, the reasons for nurses leaving the profession have been complex, arising from a range of social, economic, professional, and systemic factors.

To appreciate the depth of nursing attrition, the reader must consider the evolution of nursing as both an art and a science, as well as a career path often faced with challenges. According to Pfettscher (2021), from its origins in the era of Florence Nightingale, when nursing was formalised as a distinct vocation, to the modern complexities of highly specialised healthcare systems, the pressures faced by nurses have been persistent and multifaceted. These pressures are not confined to the workplace; they are deeply embedded with societal issues such as gender norms, economic disparities, and shifting public attitudes towards health and caregiving (NHS England, 2018).

Exploring the historical context also requires examining the systemic factors that have shaped nurses' work environments and their decisions to remain in or leave the profession. Workforce shortages, inadequate compensation, burnout, and the often overlooked emotional strain of caregiving are not recent phenomena but are challenges with historical precedence. These issues have been compounded by broader trends, including wars, pandemics, and periods of economic instability, which have tested the resilience of the nursing workforce time and again.

In this chapter, we investigate the constraints that have driven nursing attrition across different eras, shedding light on the continued struggles faced by nurses and the systemic reforms needed to address these challenges. By understanding the historical foundations of nursing attrition, we can better appreciate its ongoing impact and identify strategies to build a sustainable and supportive future for the nursing profession.

Early Development of Nursing and Initial Attrition Trends

Nineteenth-century modern nursing was formalised by key figures such as Florence Nightingale and started growing as a structured profession. "I never gave or took any excuse" is a famous quote by Florence Nightingale.

Early nurses worked in challenging conditions with long hours, low pay, and limited societal respect.

Attrition began to occur due to poor working conditions as well as high physical and emotional demands without adequate support. There were also the social stigmas, whereby nursing was seen as a lower-status job, deterring individuals from long-term commitment.

There were also wartime pressures; nurses during the Crimean War and World War II often left due to trauma, injury, or exhaustion.

The early decades of the 20th century demonstrated a more formalised route into nursing which was linked to hospitals; however, burnout was common due to poor work–life balance and hierarchical structures.

Attrition started to increase during times of economic hardship, such as the Great Depression when wages for nurses declined further. The level of attrition was evident for years until the post–World War II boom. This era started to see an increased demand for healthcare services, especially with advancements in medical technology and the rise of hospital systems. One of the challenges at the time was that many nurses left the profession due to gendered expectations. Women were often expected to leave work upon marriage or childbirth, creating a high turnover of nursing staff.

Introduction of Evidence-Based Practice Circa 1950s

The introduction of evidence-based practice (EBP) in the 1950s marked a critical moment in nursing, creating professional pathways for nurses to engage in education and research. This shift not only transformed nursing education but also elevated expectations placed on nursing students. Over time, the emphasis on EBP has redefined the nursing profession, requiring a strong foundation in critical thinking, research, and academic rigor (Cullum et al., 1997).

While this evolution has advanced the quality of patient care and the professionalisation of nursing, it has also introduced challenges. The heightened academic and clinical demands can contribute to stress, burnout, and, ultimately, attrition among nursing students. By connecting the historical origins of EBP to current trends, we can better understand how its integration into nursing curricula has influenced the profession, including its unintended impact on the retention of future nurses.

EBP in the 1950s was a transformative milestone in nursing, creating pathways for nurses to actively participate in both education and research. By integrating systematic research findings into clinical decision-making, EBP allowed nursing to move beyond tradition and intuition, establishing it as a rigorous, scientifically grounded profession. As Cullum et al. (1997) suggest, this shift redefined the expectations placed on nursing professionals, stimulating a transformation in nursing education that necessitated a strong emphasis on critical thinking, research skills, and academic rigor.

The emphasis on EBP has directly contributed to the improvement of patient care by advancing practices that are supported by research evidence rather than anecdotal or routine practices. This shift has professionalised nursing, ensuring that interventions are safer, more effective, and tailored to patients' needs. Furthermore, EBP equips nurses with the tools to adapt to rapidly evolving healthcare environments, contributing to better health outcomes, cost efficiency, and interdisciplinary collaboration.

The introduction of EBP in the 1950s was undoubtedly transformative, redefining nursing as a rigorous, research-driven profession and elevating the standards of patient care. However, this paradigm shift has also had unintended consequences that have contributed to the attrition of nurses during this period. Understanding the connection between EBP's integration and nurse retention highlights the dual impact of this development on the profession.

ACADEMIC AND CLINICAL EXPECTATIONS

The integration of EBP demanded a significant shift in nursing education, placing greater emphasis on academic rigor, critical thinking, and research skills. While this enhanced the professional standing of nursing, it also created more intensive academic and clinical training pathways. Nursing students were required to master not only foundational clinical skills but also the ability to evaluate and apply research findings in real-world scenarios. These heightened expectations placed considerable pressure on students, who faced the dual burden of maintaining academic excellence and navigating complex, evidence-informed clinical environments.

For many, the resulting stress was a significant factor in burnout and, ultimately, attrition. Those unable to meet these demands or lacking adequate support systems were at higher risk of abandoning their training or leaving the profession altogether. The increased focus on research and critical thinking, while essential for improving patient care, inadvertently created barriers for students struggling to balance these demands with personal and financial challenges (Schaufeli et al., 2017).

STRESS AND BURNOUT

The professionalisation of nursing through EBP also redefined the role of practising nurses, necessitating continuous learning and adaptation to evidence-based protocols. This shift added variables of complexity to their daily responsibilities. As Melnyk et al. (2014, p. 16) highlight, 'EBP is a problem-solving approach to the delivery of healthcare that integrates the best evidence from well-designed studies with a clinician's expertise and patient preferences.' Consequently, in addition to delivering patient care, nurses were now expected to stay updated on the latest research, critically appraise studies, and apply findings to their practice.

This incessant demand for growth and adaptation, often under resource-constrained conditions, led to widespread stress and burnout among nurses. As Aiken et al. (2002, p. 193) assert, 'higher patient-to-nurse ratios are associated with higher levels of burnout and job dissatisfaction,' highlighting the pressures faced by nursing staff. As a result, many experienced physical and emotional exhaustion, dissatisfaction with their roles, and diminished job performance. Over time, these factors contributed to the departure of nurses from the workforce, exacerbating staffing shortages and increasing the workload for those who remained. This created what describe as 'a cycle of stress and attrition, where increased demands without adequate support lead to burnout and eventual workforce depletion.'

IMPACT ON RETENTION

The professional pathways created by EBP inadvertently set a higher bar for both students and practising nurses, resulting in a more demanding environment that not all could sustain. Students struggling to meet academic demands or manage the stress of clinical training were more likely to drop out, whereas Schaufeli et al. (2017) observed that practising nurses facing chronic burnout left the profession in search of less taxing careers. Additionally, the shift to EBP highlighted disparities in institutional support, with some facilities failing to provide adequate resources for research, continuing education, or mental health support.

By linking the historical origins of EBP to contemporary challenges, it becomes evident that the evolution of nursing education and practice has been both a boon and a burden. While EBP has undoubtedly elevated the profession, its implementation has placed substantial demands on nurses, contributing to attrition. These challenges persist today (Costello, 2023), emphasising the need for comprehensive support systems, such as mentorship programmes, mental health resources, and flexible education pathways, to sustain and grow the nursing workforce.

While EBP has advanced nursing as a science-based profession and improved patient care quality, it has also contributed to attrition among nurses due to heightened expectations, stress, and burnout. Addressing these issues requires an understanding of EBP's impact and a commitment to fostering environments that balance professional excellence with well-being.

EDUCATION AND PROFESSIONAL IMPLICATIONS

The integration of EBP into nursing curricula has brought significant changes to nursing education. According to Melnyk et al. (2014), 'evidence-based practice is a problem-solving approach to clinical decision-making that integrates the best available evidence with clinical expertise and patient values.' As a result, students are now expected to understand complex research methodologies, critically appraise studies, and apply findings to clinical practice. This academic rigor has advanced a new generation of nurses who are not only practitioners but also contributors to research and healthcare innovation.

However, these advancements come with challenges. The increased expectations and demands can create stress for nursing students, who must balance intensive academic and clinical workloads. As Pulido-Martos et al. (2012, p. 19) noted, 'nursing students experience high levels of stress due to academic pressure, clinical performance, and the emotional burden of patient care.' The pressure to excel in evidence-based learning environments can exacerbate stress and contribute to mental health challenges such as burnout, a known precursor to attrition (Rudman & Gustavsson, 2012).

CHALLENGES AND RETENTION

While EBP enhances the profession's standing and the quality of care delivered, its integration into nursing education inadvertently impacts retention. As Craig and Stevens (2012, p. 74) noted, 'the rigorous demands of evidence-based practice education can contribute to academic stress, which may influence student retention rates.' The heightened academic and clinical requirements often result in a demanding educational journey. Students who struggle to meet these standards may feel overwhelmed, potentially leading to dropout rates that threaten the nursing workforce channel. Addressing this challenge requires a deeper understanding of how EBP-driven curricula affect students' experiences and implementation of strategies to mitigate these unintended consequences.

Connecting the historical origins of EBP to current trends provides valuable insights into its dual role as a transformative force and a source of stress within the profession. According to Aiken et al. (2014, p. 12), 'nursing education must strike a balance between academic rigor and student well-being to ensure both competence and workforce sustainability.' By acknowledging the challenges associated with its integration, educators and policymakers can adopt strategies to support nursing students. For instance, incorporating resilience training, mentorship programmes, and mental health resources into nursing education can help students to navigate the academic and clinical demands of EBP-centred curricula. Moreover, studies suggest that 'flexible learning pathways and institutional support can improve student retention and overall satisfaction in nursing programs' (Sitzman & Ely, 2010, p. 203). Furthermore, creating flexible pathways and promoting a culture that balances excellence with well-being may help to improve retention rates.

In conclusion, the introduction of EBP has been a cornerstone of nursing's evolution, enhancing care quality and professional identity. However, its integration into education and practice has also highlighted the need for supportive measures to sustain the nursing workforce. As Duchscher (2009, p. 105) emphasises, 'the transition from nursing education to practice is complex and requires structured support to prevent burnout and attrition.' By addressing the challenges posed, the profession can continue to advance while ensuring the well-being and success of future nurses.

Changes in the 1960s and 1970s

The feminist movement and improved workplace rights began shifting societal expectations; however, systemic issues such as unequal pay and lack of autonomy in the profession persisted. Attrition often resulted from dissatisfaction with rigid hospital hierarchies and limited career development (Lester, 2021).

The mid-20th century marked a period of societal transformation, with movements like feminism and advocacy for workplace rights driving significant changes in many professions, including nursing. These shifts challenged traditional societal norms and began reshaping women's roles in the workforce. However, despite progress, systemic barriers such as unequal pay, lack of professional autonomy, and dissatisfaction with rigid workplace hierarchies persisted in nursing, contributing to high attrition rates within the profession. Understanding these factors provides insight into the challenges faced by nurses during this transformative era and gives an indication of the broader dynamics that influenced workforce retention.

THE FEMINIST MOVEMENT AND CHANGING SOCIETAL EXPECTATIONS

The feminist movement of the mid-20th century (1940–1969) was instrumental in advancing gender equality in the workplace. Women began to advocate for better wages, workplace rights, and the dismantling of traditional gender roles that had long confined them to subordinate positions (Melchior, 2004). In nursing, these societal shifts initially raised hopes for improved professional recognition and working conditions. Nurses, predominantly women, saw the movement as an opportunity to challenge inequities that had been deeply ingrained in healthcare systems.

Despite this momentum, progress in nursing was slow. The profession remained rooted in traditional, often patriarchal structures, which limited the scope of change. While women in other fields began to gain more equitable pay and career advancement opportunities, nurses continued to grapple with systemic issues that hindered their professional autonomy and career growth.

While the feminist movement brought attention to workplace inequities, it also inspired advocacy within the nursing profession. As Evans (2004, p. 46) states, 'the feminist movement provided a critical framework for nurses to challenge traditional power structures and demand professional recognition.'

Nursing leaders also began to emerge during this time, advocating for changes that aligned with the broader feminist agenda. They called for reforms in nursing education, the expansion of advanced practice roles, and the creation of pathways for nurses to take on leadership positions within healthcare organisations. As Hewitt (2007, p. 88) explains, 'the feminist influence in nursing not only advanced educational and professional opportunities but also emphasised the importance of nurses as decision-makers within healthcare systems.' These initiatives sought to address the systemic issues driving attrition and elevate the status of nursing as a profession.

SYSTEMIC ISSUES IN NURSING: UNEQUAL PAY AND LIMITED CAREER DEVELOPMENT

One of the most pervasive challenges for nurses during this era was unequal pay. Despite their essential contributions to healthcare, nurses were often compensated far less than their male counterparts in similarly skilled professions. This disparity not only reflected broader societal undervaluation of women's work but also reinforced the perception that nursing was a subservient role within the medical hierarchy.

In addition to wage disparities, career development opportunities in nursing were limited. Hospital hierarchies often restricted nurses to roles that emphasised obedience to physicians rather than independent decision-making. Advanced educational opportunities and leadership positions were scarce, leaving many nurses feeling stagnant in their careers. For those seeking greater professional fulfilment, these systemic barriers often proved insurmountable, prompting them to leave the profession entirely.

Shaw et al. (2024) highlight that the issues of limited career development leading to attrition of nurses remains an issue today.

RIGID HOSPITAL HIERARCHIES AND WORKPLACE DISSATISFACTION

The hospital environment of the mid-20th century was characterised by rigid hierarchies that placed nurses in subordinate roles to physicians and administrators. These hierarchies perpetuated a culture of control and compliance, where nurses were expected to carry out orders rather than contribute to decision-making. This lack of autonomy was a source of significant frustration for many nurses, who felt that their expertise and judgement were undervalued.

The hierarchical structure also contributed to a workplace culture that offered little flexibility or recognition for the challenges that nurses faced. Long hours, high patient loads, and limited support from management exacerbated job dissatisfaction. For nurses who sought more collaborative and empowering work environments, these conditions were a major factor in their decision to leave the profession.

BURNOUT AND ATTRITION IN NURSING

The challenges associated with unequal pay, lack of autonomy, and rigid workplace structures often led to burnout, a condition characterised by emotional exhaustion, depersonalisation, and reduced personal accomplishment. Burnout among nurses was particularly prevalent due to the physically and emotionally demanding nature of their work, coupled with limited resources and support.

This era also saw significant workforce shortages in healthcare, which further exacerbated the pressures on nurses. With fewer colleagues to share the workload, many nurses faced overwhelming demands that made it difficult to maintain a healthy work–life balance. As a result, attrition rates soared, leaving hospitals and healthcare systems struggling to retain experienced nursing staff.

BROADER IMPACTS OF ATTRITION ON HEALTHCARE

The high attrition rates in nursing during this era had significant implications for the healthcare system. Workforce shortages strained hospitals, leading to increased patient-to-nurse ratios and compromised quality of care. The departure of experienced nurses also created gaps in institutional knowledge and mentorship, which were essential for training new nurses.

Additionally, the loss of nursing talent reinforced the perception of nursing as a high-turnover, low-satisfaction profession. This perception discouraged potential recruits from entering the field, further perpetuating workforce challenges and undermining efforts to professionalise nursing.

PROGRESS AND PERSISTENT CHALLENGES

Although the mid-20th century was a challenging time for nurses, it also marked the beginning of important changes that would shape the future of the profession. The advocacy efforts sparked by the feminist movement and nursing leaders eventually led to advancements in workplace rights, educational opportunities, and professional recognition. Over time, these changes began to address some of the systemic issues that had driven attrition, leading the way for a more equitable and sustainable nursing workforce.

However, many of the challenges that emerged during this era, such as burnout, workload pressures, and the undervaluation of nursing, continue to affect the profession today. Addressing these issues requires a sustained commitment to improving workplace conditions, enabling professional development, and ensuring equitable pay for nurses.

Late 20th Century: Professionalisation Versus Systemic Stress

Evidence from the 1980s and 1990s demonstrated that efforts were made to professionalise nursing through advanced education. According to Rafferty (1996, p. 56), 'the drive towards professionalisation in nursing was heavily influenced by the need for higher education and structured career pathways.' Changes to nurse qualifications from enrolled nurse to conversion to registered nurse reflected this shift, and registered nurses were unable to develop further unless they pursued additional qualifications, such as the 18-month midwife route, mental health nursing, or learning disabilities nursing. The eventual introduction of Project 2000 and the Diploma in Nursing marked a pivotal moment in nursing education reform. As the United Kingdom Central Council for Nursing, Midwifery and Health Visiting (UKCC) highlighted, 'Project 2000 sought to move nursing education into higher education institutions, fostering a more academically rigorous approach to training and professional development' (UKCC, 1999, p. 14).

Throughout the period of change to the nurse entry route, healthcare systems increasingly focused on cost-cutting measures, leading to staff shortages and fewer nurses to manage heavier workloads. As Aiken et al. (2002, p. 198) noted, 'understaffing and increased workloads in hospitals have been directly linked to nurse burnout, job dissatisfaction, and higher patient mortality rates.' Burnout from emotional and physical exhaustion drove many nurses out of the profession. Research by McVicar (2003, p. 63) further confirms that 'workplace stressors such as staffing shortages, extended shifts, and emotional demands contribute significantly to burnout among nurses, ultimately impacting retention.'

The 1980s and 1990s were transformative decades for the nursing profession, marked by significant efforts to professionalise nursing through advanced education and changes to qualification pathways. These efforts aimed to elevate the status of nursing and ensure that nurses were better equipped to meet the demands of increasingly complex healthcare systems. However, this period of change was also characterised by challenges, including cost-cutting measures, staffing shortages, and rising workloads, all of which contributed to burnout and attrition within the nursing workforce.

PROFESSIONALISATION OF NURSING THROUGH EDUCATION

During this period, the landscape of nursing qualifications underwent significant reform. Historically, many nurses entered the profession as enrolled nurses, a role that required less training and offered fewer opportunities for advancement. As Watson (1995, p. 26) noted, 'the enrolled nurse role, while valuable, often functioned within a restrictive scope of practice, limiting career mobility and professional recognition.' Transitioning to registered nurse status required additional training, but for much of the 1980s and early 1990s, career progression was limited unless nurses pursued specialised pathways such as the 18-month midwifery route, mental health nursing, or learning disabilities nursing. These routes offered some opportunities for specialisation, but they also required significant time and financial investment, which were not accessible to all nurses.

The introduction of Project 2000 in the late 1980s and early 1990s marked a watershed moment in nursing education. This initiative sought to standardise nursing qualifications and elevate the profession by replacing traditional hospital-based training with university-led education programmes. According to the UKCC (1986, p. 15), 'Project 2000 was designed to establish nursing as an intellectual discipline, integrating academic study with clinical practice to produce critically thinking practitioners.' Under Project 2000, nursing students earned a Diploma in Nursing, which emphasised academic rigor alongside clinical training. This shift aligned nursing with other professional disciplines, highlighting the importance of theoretical knowledge and critical thinking in addition to practical skills.

Project 2000 aimed to address long-standing issues within the profession, including inconsistent training standards and the lack of recognition for nursing as an academic discipline. As Maggs (1996, p. 5) explains, 'one of the primary motivations behind Project 2000 was to bridge the gap between the vocational nature of nursing and the growing complexity of healthcare demands.' By emphasising higher education, the initiative sought to prepare nurses for the increasingly complex demands of modern healthcare and to position nursing as a respected and autonomous profession.

CHALLENGES OF CHANGE: WORKFORCE SHORTAGES AND COST-CUTTING MEASURES

While the changes introduced by Project 2000 and other educational reforms were designed to benefit the nursing profession, they coincided with significant challenges in the broader healthcare system. During the 1980s and 1990s, many countries, particularly in the Western world, experienced economic pressures that led to widespread cost-cutting measures in healthcare. As Stokes (1999) observed, 'economic constraints and austerity measures significantly impacted healthcare systems, leading to reduced funding for staffing and resources.' Hospitals and health systems faced mounting financial constraints, resulting in staff reductions and hiring freezes.

These measures had a direct impact on nursing. With fewer nurses employed, those who remained in the workforce were required to manage increasingly heavy workloads. According to Aiken et al. (2002), 'nurse staffing reductions and increased patient-to-nurse ratios were directly linked to diminished quality of care, job dissatisfaction, and increased burnout among nurses.' This strain was exacerbated by the growing complexity of patient care, as advances in medical technology and treatments created new demands on healthcare providers. Nurses were often expected to perform tasks that extended beyond their traditional roles, contributing to a sense of being overburdened and undervalued. As Laschinger et al. (2001) highlighted, 'increased role ambiguity and responsibility without corresponding authority or recognition is a significant factor contributing to nursing burnout.'

Additionally, the shift to university-based education under Project 2000 created a temporary disruption in the supply of newly qualified nurses. As Maggs (1996) pointed out, 'the transition from hospital-based to university-based education was designed to elevate nursing's academic status but also created a short-term gap in workforce numbers as fewer nurses entered the profession during the transition period.' The transition from hospital-based training to academic institutions meant that fewer nurses were entering the workforce during the implementation period, further compounding staffing shortages.

THE IMPACT OF BURNOUT ON THE NURSING WORKFORCE

The combination of heavier workloads, staffing shortages, and the emotional demands of nursing contributed to widespread burnout among nurses during this era. Burnout, characterised by emotional exhaustion, depersonalisation, and a reduced sense of personal accomplishment, became a significant factor driving nurses out of the profession.

Physical and emotional exhaustion was particularly acute in settings such as emergency departments, intensive care units, and long-term care facilities, where patient needs were most urgent and staffing levels were often inadequate. Nurses in these environments frequently reported feeling overwhelmed, unsupported, and unable to provide the level of care they believed their patients deserved. This disconnect between professional expectations and the realities of the workplace led many nurses to experience moral distress, further contributing to burnout and attrition.

For some nurses, the demanding nature of nursing became untenable, leading them to leave the profession altogether. This exodus created a vicious cycle: as more nurses left the workforce, those who remained faced even greater workloads, intensifying the pressures that had driven their colleagues to leave.

THE BROADER IMPLICATIONS OF ATTRITION

The high rates of attrition during the 1980s and 1990s had far-reaching implications for healthcare systems. Staffing shortages compromised the quality of patient care, with fewer nurses available to meet patients' needs. In many cases, this led to longer wait times, higher patient-to-nurse ratios, and reduced access to care, particularly in underserved communities.

The loss of experienced nurses also created gaps in institutional knowledge and mentorship, making it more challenging to train and support newly qualified nurses entering the workforce. These challenges undermined the goals of initiatives like Project 2000, which sought to elevate the profession and improve patient outcomes through advanced education and training.

PROGRESS AMIDST CHALLENGES

Despite these challenges, the changes introduced during the 1980s and 1990s laid the groundwork for many of the advancements seen in nursing today. The shift to university-based education under Project 2000 helped to establish nursing as an academic discipline, fostering a new generation of nurses with a strong foundation in EBP, research, and critical thinking.

Moreover, the emphasis on advanced education created pathways for nurses to pursue specialised roles and leadership positions, gradually breaking down some of the barriers to career progression that had limited the profession in the past. Over time, these changes contributed to a more empowered and professional nursing workforce, even as the challenges of burnout and attrition continued to pose significant obstacles.

ECONOMIC AND POLICY SHIFTS

The Impact of Hospital Mergers, Budget Cuts, and Managed Care on Nurses

The healthcare landscape underwent significant transformation in the latter part of the 20th century (1970–1999), with hospital mergers, budget cuts, and the rise of managed care reshaping the way healthcare was delivered. While these changes were intended to streamline services and reduce costs, they had a profound and often negative impact on the nursing workforce. Nurses, who are at the heart of patient care, were heavily affected by these structural shifts, leading to increased job insecurity, stress, and dissatisfaction. As McClure and Hinshaw (2002, p. 22) highlight, 'nurses' job satisfaction and overall well-being were deeply impacted by the organisational changes that came with mergers and the expansion of managed care.' The reliance on part-time or agency nurses became a particularly prominent factor in these challenges, further contributing to an already strained workforce. According to Hayes (2004, p. 91), 'the increasing use of part-time and agency nurses has been linked to diminished continuity of care, lower team cohesion, and an overall decline in staff morale.'

In the 1980s and 1990s, many hospitals underwent mergers as part of efforts to streamline operations, reduce overhead costs, and consolidate resources in response to increasing financial pressures. The idea behind these mergers was to improve efficiency and provide a more coordinated system of care. However, for nurses, hospital mergers often led to job losses, changes in working conditions, and diminished morale. According to Stone (2001, p. 317), 'hospital mergers, while financially motivated, often resulted in layoffs and role consolidation, leading to increased job insecurity among nurses.'

As hospitals merged, many nurses faced job insecurity due to reductions in staff. Mergers typically resulted in duplications of roles, and many nursing positions were either eliminated or consolidated. Nurses found themselves in competition for fewer roles, and seniority was sometimes disregarded in favour of cost-cutting measures. The resulting layoffs or position eliminations caused considerable uncertainty among nurses, particularly for those who had long-standing careers at hospitals that were now part of a larger health system. This job insecurity not only increased stress but also contributed to high attrition rates as nurses sought more stable employment opportunities elsewhere. Aiken et al. (2002, p. 199) argue that 'job insecurity is a known precursor to burnout and job dissatisfaction, contributing to attrition in the nursing profession.'

Additionally, the restructuring that often accompanied hospital mergers led to significant changes in work practices. Nurses faced longer shifts, heavier patient loads, and a reduced ability to form strong working relationships with colleagues. These changes were not always accompanied by adequate training or support, which further heightened stress levels. As Laschinger et al. (2001, p. 78) assert, 'poor organisational support during periods of change exacerbates stress, leading to emotional exhaustion and a decline in job satisfaction.' Nurses, who were already dealing with high levels of emotional and physical exhaustion, found themselves overwhelmed by the demands of an increasingly impersonal and bureaucratic healthcare environment.

Budget Cuts and Their Effect on Nursing Workloads

Budget cuts in healthcare institutions were another major factor that contributed to nurse dissatisfaction during this period. In response to rising healthcare costs, many hospitals and health systems implemented significant reductions in spending. These cuts often targeted nursing staff, leading to reductions in nursing hours, salary freezes, and the elimination of critical support staff.

With fewer resources available to support them, nurses were forced to take on heavier patient loads and perform additional administrative duties that previously would have been handled by other departments. The pressure to provide high-quality care with fewer resources led to a strained and sometimes unsafe work environment. Nurses, already working long hours, were often expected to care for more patients than was advisable, increasing the risk of burnout and fatigue. According to Aiken et al. (2002, p. 199), 'nurses working in understaffed environments are more likely to experience fatigue, burnout, and emotional exhaustion, which in turn compromise patient care.'

The physical demands of the job, combined with the emotional toll of providing care in underresourced settings, caused many nurses to question their ability to maintain their commitment to their patients and their profession. Nurses, who had traditionally played a central role in patient care, found themselves relegated to more routine tasks as hospitals shifted to more cost-effective practices. For example, in many instances, nurses were asked to perform more administrative duties, such as completing paperwork and handling logistical tasks, in an effort to reduce the need for clerical staff. This shift in responsibilities, combined with increased patient workloads, led to feelings of dissatisfaction among nurses who felt that their roles as caregivers were being undermined. As McGillis Hall et al. (2007, p. 59) stated, 'the shift from direct patient care to administrative tasks diminishes nurses' professional satisfaction and undermines their sense of purpose in the workplace.'

Nurses were heavily affected by hospital mergers, budget cuts, and the rise of managed care. An increase in reliance on part-time or agency nurses contributed to job insecurity and dissatisfaction.

The Rise of Managed Care and Its Impact on Nurses

The rise of managed care in the 1990s added another layer of complexity to the challenges faced by nurses. Managed care, which aimed to reduce healthcare costs by limiting access to services and controlling the use of medical resources, introduced policies and structures that often conflicted with nurses' professional values. Managed care organisations focused on controlling costs and improving efficiency, frequently at the expense of patient-centred care.

For nurses, this meant that they were increasingly asked to make decisions based on cost considerations rather than patient needs. The emphasis on efficiency led to more standardised care protocols that left little room for clinical judgement or individual patient needs. Nurses were required to follow strict guidelines that were often dictated by administrators rather than based on the individual care requirements of patients. This lack of autonomy over clinical decision-making created frustration and dissatisfaction among nurses, who felt that their professional expertise was being undermined.

Furthermore, managed care organisations often imposed unrealistic patient care ratios. Nurses found themselves caring for more patients than was safe, which not only compromised patient safety but also contributed to a sense of helplessness and emotional exhaustion. As nurses struggled to meet these demands, they experienced high levels of stress, burnout, and job dissatisfaction.

The Increasing Reliance on Part-Time and Agency Nurses

As hospital systems and healthcare institutions sought to manage their budgets, many turned to part-time or agency nurses to fill staffing gaps. The reliance on these workers was seen as a cost-saving measure, as hospitals could hire temporary staff without providing benefits or long-term employment commitments. While part-time and agency nurses played a vital role in keeping hospitals staffed, their presence often exacerbated the challenges faced by full-time nurses.

Part-time and agency nurses, while offering flexibility to healthcare systems, contributed to feelings of job insecurity among full-time nursing staff. The increasing use of temporary workers meant that full-time nurses were often asked to train or work alongside agency nurses, many of whom lacked the institutional knowledge or experience that full-time staff possessed. This created tension within nursing teams, as experienced nurses felt that the quality of care was compromised when less-experienced staff members were utilised to fill gaps in care delivery.

The use of agency nurses further destabilised the workforce. Agency nurses, who were often paid more than their full-time peers, created a perception of inequality and frustration among the regular nursing staff. Full-time nurses, who were often working under stressful conditions, felt that their contributions were undervalued, as temporary workers were given higher pay for the same tasks. This disparity further fuelled dissatisfaction and resentment among nurses, contributing to a toxic work environment and higher turnover rates.

JOB INSECURITY AND ITS LONG-TERM EFFECTS

The cumulative effects of hospital mergers, budget cuts, the rise of managed care, and the increased reliance on part-time and agency nurses led to widespread job insecurity in the nursing profession. Nurses were no longer able to rely on stable, long-term employment, and the lack of job security became a driving force behind high attrition rates. This insecurity not only affected nurses' mental and emotional well-being but also hindered their ability to provide the quality of care that patients needed and deserved.

The lack of stability in the workforce, combined with rising levels of stress and dissatisfaction, resulted in a significant number of experienced nurses leaving the profession. Many nurses found themselves questioning the value of their work in an environment that prioritised cost cutting and efficiency over patient care. As a result, healthcare institutions faced ongoing difficulties in maintaining a stable, experienced nursing workforce.

The 21st Century: Ongoing Challenges and New Pressures

THE GLOBAL NURSING SHORTAGE AND ITS IMPACT ON ATTRITION RATES: A PRE- AND POST-COVID-19 ANALYSIS

Nursing has long been regarded as the backbone of healthcare systems worldwide, yet it faces numerous challenges, particularly when it comes to staffing shortages and attrition rates. According to Farahani et al. (2024) the nursing shortage was a well-documented issue even before the onset of the COVID-19 pandemic. However, the pandemic significantly exacerbated these challenges, leading to a surge in attrition rates and further straining already fragile healthcare systems. The global nursing shortage, fuelled by various factors such as ageing populations, increasing healthcare demands, and systemic issues within the profession, has become one of the most critical concerns in healthcare globally.

This section explores the historical context of nursing shortages, the factors contributing to the current crisis, and the effects of the COVID-19 pandemic on nursing retention. By analysing global trends, we can better understand the reasons behind nursing attrition and its implications for healthcare systems worldwide.

THE PREPANDEMIC NURSING SHORTAGE: HISTORICAL CONTEXT AND CONTRIBUTING FACTORS

Before the COVID-19 pandemic, the global nursing shortage was already a growing issue. Several factors contributed to this shortage, including demographic shifts, increasing healthcare demands, and poor working conditions. One of the most significant drivers of the nursing shortage has been the ageing population in many countries. As populations across the world have aged, the demand for healthcare services has risen exponentially, placing immense pressure on healthcare systems. Older adults typically require more frequent and intensive medical care, increasing the burden on healthcare workers, particularly nurses, who often provide the majority of direct patient care.

At the same time, many developed countries, such as those in Europe, North America, and parts of Asia, were experiencing an ageing nursing workforce. As older nurses began to retire, there were not enough younger nurses entering the profession to replace them. This demographic imbalance created a gap between the supply and demand for nursing services, which worsened the overall shortage.

In addition to demographic factors, there were systemic issues within the profession itself that contributed to the nursing shortage. Nurses often cited poor staffing ratios, inadequate pay, and lack of professional development opportunities as reasons for leaving the profession. Inadequate staffing ratios were particularly problematic, leading to increased workloads and burnout. Nurses were frequently tasked with managing more patients than they could reasonably care for, which compromised patient care quality and contributed to feelings of stress and exhaustion among nursing staff.

Inadequate support in the workplace, both from management and colleagues, was another significant factor that led to high attrition rates. Many nurses reported feeling undervalued and overburdened as hospitals and healthcare institutions struggled to provide the necessary resources and support. The lack of proper staffing, training, and mental health resources created an environment where nurses felt unsupported, which in turn led to high levels of dissatisfaction and burnout.

THE COVID-19 PANDEMIC: EXACERBATING THE NURSING SHORTAGE

While the nursing shortage was already a pressing issue, the onset of the COVID-19 pandemic in 2020 further exacerbated the crisis. The pandemic placed an overwhelming burden on healthcare systems around the world, leading to unprecedented challenges for nurses. The nursing workforce, already stretched thin, faced an onslaught of new and complex demands as healthcare facilities struggled to cope with the surge of COVID-19 cases.

Nurses were on the front lines of the pandemic, often working long hours in high-stress environments, dealing with critically ill patients, and facing the emotional toll of patient death. The physical demands of caring for COVID-19 patients, combined with the psychological stress, took a significant toll on nurses' well-being. Many nurses reported experiencing anxiety, depression, and posttraumatic stress disorder (PTSD) as a result of the constant exposure to death and suffering. The mental and emotional strain, compounded by physical exhaustion, led many nurses to reconsider their careers or leave the profession altogether.

In addition to the direct stressors of patient care, the pandemic disrupted healthcare systems in other ways. Hospitals were forced to implement strict infection control measures, leading to increased isolation of patients and a lack of personal protective equipment (PPE) for healthcare workers. Nurses were often required to work in unfamiliar and unsafe conditions, further contributing to burnout and job dissatisfaction.

Moreover, the rapid spread of COVID-19 led to widespread staffing shortages, as many nurses fell ill or were required to quarantine. This created a vicious cycle in which the existing nursing workforce had to take on even greater responsibilities, leading to increased workloads, further burnout, and more nurses leaving the profession. In some countries the shortage became so severe that healthcare systems had to rely on temporary international nurses, which only provided a short-term solution to a long-term problem.

CONTRIBUTING FACTORS TO NURSING ATTRITION DURING THE PANDEMIC

Nurses have long faced issues related to poor working conditions, but the pandemic highlighted these challenges in detail. According to Farahani et al. (2024), nurses frequently cited poor staffing ratios, inadequate support, and burnout as the primary reasons for leaving the profession. The increased workload caused by the pandemic exacerbated these issues, and many nurses reported feeling unsupported by healthcare institutions and government policies:

1. *Poor Staffing Ratios*: As healthcare systems were overwhelmed by the pandemic, the shortage of nurses led to even higher patient-to-nurse ratios. Nurses were often tasked with caring for more patients than was safe or manageable, which increased stress levels and reduced the quality of care. The intense pressure to care for critically ill patients, combined with the absence of sufficient support staff, led to physical and emotional exhaustion among nurses.
2. *Inadequate Support*: Many nurses reported feeling unsupported by their employers during the pandemic. Healthcare systems were stretched to their limits, and nurses often had to cope with inadequate resources, including PPE

and mental health support. Nurses were frequently exposed to high levels of stress without the appropriate coping mechanisms or support systems in place, leading to burnout and attrition.

3. *Burnout*: The combination of high patient loads, emotional distress, and physical exhaustion contributed to widespread burnout among nurses. Burnout is characterised by feelings of emotional exhaustion, depersonalisation, and a reduced sense of personal accomplishment. During the pandemic, burnout rates among nurses skyrocketed, with many nurses experiencing significant emotional and mental health challenges. This burnout, coupled with job dissatisfaction, led to higher turnover rates and an accelerated exodus from the profession.

LONG-TERM EFFECTS ON THE GLOBAL NURSING WORKFORCE

The effects of the COVID-19 pandemic on the global nursing workforce have been profound. The pandemic exacerbated an already fragile nursing workforce, leading to increased attrition rates, decreased retention, and a worsening shortage of nurses. As noted by Duffield et al. (2020, p. 6), 'the COVID-19 pandemic has amplified the pre-existing vulnerabilities in the nursing workforce, contributing to higher rates of burnout and attrition.' As the demand for healthcare services continues to rise, particularly in light of ageing populations and ongoing health crises, the nursing shortage remains a critical issue. Aiken et al. (2021, p. 105) further highlight that 'the pandemic has intensified the global shortage of nurses, with many leaving the profession due to physical and emotional exhaustion, leading to a crisis in healthcare systems worldwide.'

Efforts to address the nursing shortage must focus on both short-term solutions and long-term strategies. In the short term, healthcare systems must focus on providing better support for nurses, including improved staffing ratios, adequate PPE, and access to mental health resources. Shanafelt et al. (2020, p. 213) emphasise that 'supporting the mental health and well-being of healthcare workers during crises is essential not only to reduce burnout but also to maintain retention and ensure the quality of patient care.' Addressing burnout and improving workplace conditions will be critical to retaining existing nurses and preventing further attrition. Buerhaus et al. (2020, p. 4) argue that 'addressing the psychological and emotional well-being of nurses is crucial in mitigating burnout and improving retention in the healthcare sector.'

In the long term, there must be a concerted effort to increase the number of nurses entering the profession. This will require investments in nursing education, better incentives for young people to pursue nursing careers, and policies that promote career development and job satisfaction for nurses. Laschinger et al. (2021, p. 78) suggest that 'investing in nursing education, creating pathways for career advancement, and fostering positive work environments are critical to building a sustainable workforce for the future.' Governments and healthcare systems must also prioritise the recruitment and retention of nurses, particularly in underserved areas, to ensure that the nursing workforce is sufficient to meet the growing demands of healthcare. Drennan et al. (2021, p. 299) highlight that 'policy changes that focus on addressing the geographic maldistribution of nurses and the promotion of nursing careers in underserved areas are critical to addressing global nursing shortages.'

INCREASED EXPOSURE TO HEALTH RISKS AND INADEQUATE PPE

A central issue during the early months of the COVID-19 pandemic was the global shortage of PPE, which placed healthcare workers at a significant risk of contracting the virus. PPE, including face masks, gowns, gloves, and face shields, is designed to protect healthcare workers from exposure to hazardous substances or infectious agents. However, the overwhelming demand for PPE during the pandemic led to significant shortages, leaving many nurses and other healthcare professionals exposed to greater health risks.

Nurses were often forced to reuse PPE or work without the necessary protective gear due to supply chain issues, budget constraints, or administrative failures. This lack of adequate protection contributed to anxiety and moral distress among nurses as they were placed in situations where they had to choose between their duty to care for patients and their own safety. Nurses reported feeling torn between wanting to provide care to their patients and fearing the possibility of becoming infected themselves or, worse, transmitting the virus to others.

The lack of PPE and the exposure to health risks further compounded the emotional and physical strain on nurses. Many nurses who were already working under intense pressure felt demoralised by the inadequate resources and support provided to them. The inability to protect themselves adequately led to feelings of fear and helplessness, which contributed to the mental health challenges many nurses faced. For some, the constant exposure to risk became unbearable, leading to a spike in attrition as nurses chose to leave their positions or even the profession entirely to protect their health and well-being.

MORAL DISTRESS AND SYSTEMIC FAILURES

Another significant factor in the spike of nursing attrition during the pandemic was the moral distress experienced by nurses. Moral distress occurs when healthcare professionals are unable to act according to their ethical beliefs because of institutional constraints, such as inadequate resources, staffing shortages, or systemic failures. The pandemic exacerbated these issues, as many nurses found themselves in situations where they could not provide the level of care they felt was necessary due to overwhelmed healthcare systems.

Nurses were frequently forced to make difficult decisions regarding patient care, often having to prioritise certain patients over others due to limited resources such as ventilators or intensive care unit beds. This created an environment of moral conflict, where nurses were unable to follow their ethical duty to provide equal care to all patients. For many, this was an emotionally devastating experience, leading to feelings of guilt and frustration. The inability to meet the expectations of both patients and their professional standards contributed to moral injury, which in turn led to increased burnout and emotional exhaustion.

Additionally, the rapid pace at which policies and procedures had to be rewritten in response to the evolving pandemic further exacerbated systemic failures within healthcare organisations. Nurses were forced to adjust to new protocols on a near-daily basis, often without sufficient training or support. This lack of clear guidance and administrative oversight made it difficult for nurses to navigate the challenges of patient care, leading to confusion, frustration, and burnout. Systemic failures, such as understaffing, lack of support for mental health, and inconsistent communication, compounded the stress that nurses experienced and contributed to high levels of attrition during the pandemic.

PTSD AND MENTAL HEALTH CHALLENGES

As a result of the intense emotional, physical, and moral strain of the pandemic, many nurses experienced PTSD, a mental health condition that can develop after exposure to traumatic events. Nurses who were on the frontlines of COVID-19 care often witnessed traumatic scenes, including mass casualties, death, and suffering. The inability to save lives and the constant exposure to patient death led to feelings of helplessness, grief, and trauma.

The experience of PTSD was compounded by the isolation that many nurses felt during the pandemic. Due to social distancing measures and strict quarantine protocols, many nurses found themselves without a strong support network. Colleagues who were also under immense stress were not always able to provide the emotional support that might have helped to alleviate some of the trauma. The stigma surrounding mental health in healthcare, coupled with the overwhelming demands of the job, made it difficult for nurses to seek the help they needed.

As PTSD and other mental health conditions began to emerge among nurses, many chose to leave the profession to protect their mental well-being. The pandemic underscored the importance of mental health support for healthcare workers, yet many nurses still felt that the resources available to them were insufficient. In many cases the systemic neglect of mental health resources in healthcare led to attrition, as nurses were left with little support to cope with the emotional toll of their work.

THE LASTING IMPACT ON NURSING ATTRITION

The spike in nursing attrition during the COVID-19 pandemic has had a lasting impact on the nursing profession. The loss of experienced and dedicated nurses has created a critical shortage of healthcare workers, further straining healthcare systems. The emotional, physical, and mental toll of the pandemic continues to affect nurses long after the peak of the crisis, with many reporting lingering feelings of burnout, trauma, and PTSD.

While efforts to recruit new nurses into the workforce are essential, it is equally important to address the root causes of attrition, including insufficient support, inadequate resources, and the lack of mental health care for healthcare workers. In the aftermath of the pandemic, healthcare systems must prioritise the well-being of their nursing staff to prevent further attrition and ensure the stability of the healthcare workforce.

Key Historical Drivers

Key historical drivers include the following:

- *Work Environment*: Poor conditions, heavy workloads, and lack of resources
- *Economic Factors*: Budget cuts, wage stagnation, and lack of job security
- *Social Expectations*: Gender norms and historical limited retention
- *Professional Challenges*: Limited career advancement and lack of autonomy
- *Systemic Crises*: Pandemics, wars, and healthcare policy changes

The historical patterns of nurse attrition reveal a persistent tension between the vital role that nurses play in heathcare and the systemic undervaluation of their work. Addressing these issues requires sustained efforts to improve working conditions, increase professional respect, and provide better support systems.

A closer look at these key drivers reveals a complex, long-standing tension between the critical role that nurses play in patient care and the systemic undervaluation of their work. To better understand nursing attrition, it is essential to explore several historical factors that have contributed to this issue, including poor work environments, economic pressures, social expectations, professional limitations, and the impact of systemic crises like pandemics and wars.

WORK ENVIRONMENT: POOR CONDITIONS, HEAVY WORKLOADS, AND LACK OF RESOURCES

The work environment has been one of the most significant drivers of nursing attrition throughout history. Nurses have long faced demanding conditions, characterised by heavy workloads, insufficient staffing, and inadequate resources. In many healthcare settings, particularly during periods of high patient volume or staffing shortages, nurses have been required to care for more patients than is safe, leading to burnout and emotional exhaustion. The work environment often lacks the necessary tools or support systems to meet the demands of patient care, resulting in an overwhelming and unsustainable workload.

These conditions were especially evident in the 19th and early 20th centuries, when nursing was seen as a largely unregulated profession with limited infrastructure. Inadequate sanitation, overcrowded hospitals, and minimal access to medical supplies or technology compounded the difficulty of nursing work. In the modern era, despite advances in medical care, understaffing continues to persist as a critical issue, leaving nurses with fewer resources to care for patients. This has led to significant levels of stress and frustration among nurses, which have contributed to their decision to leave the profession.

ECONOMIC FACTORS: BUDGET CUTS, WAGE STAGNATION, AND LACK OF JOB SECURITY

Economic factors have consistently influenced nursing attrition, particularly in relation to budget cuts, wage stagnation, and a lack of job security. Healthcare systems, especially in times of economic downturn, often face budget constraints that lead to cuts in staffing, training, and other resources necessary for effective patient care. These budget cuts result in higher workloads for nurses and inadequate compensation for their increased responsibilities.

Wage stagnation has also been a historical driver of nursing attrition. Despite the critical nature of their work, nurses have often been underpaid relative to their contributions. In many countries, wage growth in nursing has not kept pace with inflation or the rising cost of living. Furthermore, the limited opportunity for career advancement within nursing has compounded the issue. Nurses often face a "glass ceiling" in their careers, where they are unable to move into higher-paying or more prestigious roles without seeking additional, costly qualifications. This lack of economic mobility has driven many nurses to leave the profession in search of better-paying opportunities in other sectors or professions.

SOCIAL EXPECTATIONS: GENDER NORMS AND HISTORICAL LIMITED RETENTION

Social expectations, particularly gender norms, have historically played a significant role in nursing attrition. Nursing has long been considered a female-dominated profession, and the expectations placed on women in this context have shaped the profession's development. Nurses were often expected to perform emotional labour and to be self-sacrificial, which created an environment of undervaluation and limited career retention. Gendered stereotypes, such as the notion that nursing is an extension of women's 'natural' caregiving roles, led to the marginalisation of nursing as a true profession, despite its technical and intellectual demands.

Furthermore, the historical lack of retention can be attributed to the societal expectation that women would eventually leave the workforce to marry and raise children. This cyclical entry and exit from the profession limited career stability for women and reinforced the gendered nature of nursing. These social expectations created an environment where nursing was not viewed as a long-term, professional career but rather a temporary job or an extension of domestic duties.

PROFESSIONAL CHALLENGES: LIMITED CAREER ADVANCEMENT AND LACK OF AUTONOMY

Professional challenges, particularly limited career advancement and lack of autonomy, have also contributed to nursing attrition. Historically, nursing has been a hierarchical profession, with nurses often positioned at the bottom of the healthcare hierarchy, under the supervision of doctors and hospital administrators. This power imbalance has been a key driver of dissatisfaction, as nurses have had little control over their work environments or the care they provide. The lack of professional autonomy made nursing work feel less fulfilling and contributed to feelings of disempowerment among nurses.

In addition to limited autonomy, nursing has often lacked a clear path for career advancement. While there have been improvements in nursing education and opportunities for specialisation in recent years, for much of its history, nursing did not provide clear opportunities for upward mobility. Many nurses were forced to remain in staff positions without the possibility of promotion or leadership roles. As a result, nurses who sought career progression were often forced to leave the profession or pursue additional qualifications in other healthcare fields, further contributing to attrition.

SYSTEMIC CRISES: PANDEMICS, WARS, AND HEALTHCARE POLICY CHANGES

Systemic crises, such as pandemics, wars, and health policy changes, have historically played a major role in exacerbating nursing attrition. The nursing profession has been particularly vulnerable during times of crisis, as the demands on nurses increase dramatically, often without corresponding increases in support or resources. Wars, for example, have led to an influx of casualties and the need for rapid mobilisation of nursing staff. Similarly, pandemics like the 1918 influenza outbreak and the COVID-19 pandemic placed enormous strain on the nursing workforce, as nurses were often required to work long hours in unsafe, high-risk environments.

The COVID-19 pandemic, in particular, illuminated the vulnerability of the nursing profession to systemic crises. Nurses were faced with overwhelming patient numbers, inadequate PPE, and insufficient support, all of which contributed to unprecedented attrition rates. The emotional toll of the pandemic, coupled with physical exhaustion and moral distress, led many nurses to leave the profession entirely or retire early. The pandemic served as a reminder of the critical need for healthcare systems to better prepare for crises and to invest in the well-being of the nursing workforce.

Conclusion: Addressing the Historical Drivers of Nursing Attrition

The historical patterns of nursing attrition demonstrate a complex interchange between the crucial role that nurses play in healthcare and the systemic undervaluation of their work. From poor working conditions and economic pressures to gendered social expectations and professional limitations, nurses have long been faced with challenges that make it difficult to remain in the profession. These challenges have been exacerbated during times of systemic crisis, such as pandemics and wars, which place an additional strain on an already overburdened workforce (Adakpa & Costello, 2023).

Addressing these historical drivers of attrition requires a multifaceted approach that includes improving working conditions, increasing job security, and offering better career advancement opportunities. Furthermore, it is essential to challenge gender norms and societal expectations that undervalue the profession and limit nurses' ability to thrive professionally. By recognising the systemic issues that contribute to nursing attrition, healthcare systems can take meaningful steps to improve the profession, enhance retention, and ensure that nurses can continue to provide high-quality care to patients in the years to come.

This detailed examination of nursing attrition highlights several persistent historical factors that have contributed to the high turnover rates in the profession. Each of these factors, ranging from challenging work environments and economic pressures to gender norms and systemic crises, has played a significant role in the marginalisation and undervaluation of nursing work.

Summary

Work Environment: Historically, poor working conditions, insufficient staffing, and a lack of resources have created unsustainable workloads for nurses. The result has been burnout, emotional exhaustion, and, ultimately, attrition. This issue persists today despite advances in healthcare.

Economic Factors: Budget cuts, wage stagnation, and lack of job security have compounded the challenges that nurses face. Economic pressures often lead to staff reductions and increased workloads without corresponding compensation. Wage stagnation, coupled with limited career advancement, has also driven many nurses to leave for better-paying opportunities.

Social Expectations: Gender norms have long shaped nursing, with the profession being viewed as an extension of women's caregiving roles. This has led to undervaluation and limited career retention. The societal expectation that women would eventually leave the workforce for family reasons has further hindered the profession's long-term stability.

Professional Challenges: Nurses have historically had limited autonomy and career advancement opportunities. The hierarchical nature of the healthcare system has left nurses at the bottom, often without a clear path for promotion. Many have sought career advancement outside of nursing, contributing to attrition.

Systemic Crises: Events like pandemics and wars have placed additional strain on the nursing workforce, exacerbating attrition. The COVID-19 pandemic, for example, revealed vulnerabilities in the healthcare system and led to widespread burnout and early retirements among nurses.

Conclusion: Tackling the historical drivers of nursing attrition requires systemic change, including improving working conditions, offering better pay and career advancement opportunities, challenging gendered expectations, and ensuring preparedness for crises. Only by addressing these long-standing issues can healthcare systems retain the critical nursing workforce needed to provide high-quality care.

References

Adakpa, I., & Costello, A. (2023). Factors contributing to attrition – A qualitative study of undergraduate nursing students. SSRN. https://papers.ssrn.com/abstract=4771558

Aiken, L. H., Cimiotti, J. P., Sloane, D. M., Smith, H. L., Flynn, L., & Neff, D. F. (2014). The effects of nurse staffing and nurse education on patient deaths in hospitals with different nurse work environments. *Medical Care, 49*(12), 1047–1053. https://doi.org/10.1097/MLR.0b013e3182330b6e.

Aiken, L. H., Clarke, S. P., Sloane, D. M., Sochalski, J., & Silber, J. H. (2002). Hospital nurse staffing and patient mortality, nurse burnout, and job dissatisfaction. *JAMA, 288*(16), 1987–1993. https://doi.org/10.1001/jama.288.16.1987.

Aiken, L. H., Sloane, D. M., & Griffiths, P. (2021). Nursing staffing and patient outcomes: A global perspective. *International Journal of Nursing Studies, 124*, 103982. https://doi.org/10.1016/j.ijnurstu.2021.103982.

Buerhaus, P. I., Skinner, L. E., Auerbach, D. I., & Staiger, D. O. (2020). The impact of COVID-19 on the health workforce in the United States. *The New England Journal of Medicine, 383*(20), 1981–1983. https://doi.org/10.1056/NEJMp2028649.

Costello, A. (2023). *Undergraduate nurses at risk of attrition: NHS England funded project* (Unpublished project report).

Craig, J. V., & Stevens, K. R. (2012). *Evidence-based practice in nursing and healthcare: A guide to best practice.* Lippincott Williams & Wilkins.

Cullum, N., et al. (1997). Evidence-based nursing: An introduction. *Nursing Standard, 11*(28), 32–33. https://doi.org/10.7748/ns.11.28.32.s46.

Drennan, J., Grant, A., & Lethbridge, D. (2021). Addressing the global shortage of nurses: Lessons learned from COVID-19. *Journal of Nursing Regulation, 12*(1), 43–49. https://doi.org/10.1016/j.jonr.2021.01.004.

Duchscher, J. E. B. (2009). Transition shock: The initial stage of role adaptation for newly graduated registered nurses. *Journal of Advanced Nursing, 65*(5), 1103–1113. https://doi.org/10.1111/j.1365-2648.2008.04898.x.

Duffield, C. M., Roche, M. A., Blay, N., & Stasa, H. (2020). The impact of COVID-19 on the nursing workforce: A global perspective. *Journal of Nursing Management, 28*(3), 353–358. https://doi.org/10.1111/jonm.13099.

Evans, J. (2004). Men in nursing: Issues of gender segregation and hidden advantage. *Journal of Advanced Nursing, 47*(3), 321–328. https://doi.org/10.1111/j.1365-2648.2004.03096.x.

Farahani, M. A., Nargesi, S., Saniee, N., Dolatshahi, Z., Heidari Beni, F., & Shariatpanahi, S. (2024). Factors affecting nurses retention during the COVID-19 pandemic: A systematic review. *Human Resources for Health, 22*, 78. https://doi.org/10.1186/s12960-024-00960-7.

Hayes, L. J. (2004). The use of agency nurses: Impact on job satisfaction. *Journal of Nursing Administration, 34*(12), 512–520. https://doi.org/10.1097/00005110-200412000-00004.

Hewitt, J. (2007). Critical perspectives on nursing and feminism. *Nursing Inquiry, 14*(1), 21–29. https://doi.org/10.1111/j.1440-1800.2007.00348.x.

Laschinger, H. K., Finegan, J., & Shamian, J. (2001). Promoting nurses' health: Impact of workplace empowerment on burnout and quality of care. *Nursing Research, 50*(2), 55–64. https://doi.org/10.1097/00006199-200103000-00002.

Laschinger, H. K. S., Finegan, J., & Shamian, J. (2021). Creating healthier workplaces: The importance of leadership and organisational culture in nursing. *Journal of Nursing Administration, 51*(3), 122–128. https://doi.org/10.1097/NNA.0000000000001012.

Lester, L. A. (2021). The 1960s: The role of feminism and the women's movement. In *Women and the practice of medicine: A new history (1950–2020)* (pp. 25–47). Springer International Publishing.

Maggs, C. (1996). A history of nursing: A history of caring? *Journal of Advanced Nursing, 23*(6), 1130–1135. https://doi.org/10.1111/j.1365-2648.1996.tb03114.x.

McClure, M. L., & Hinshaw, A. S. (2002). Magnet hospitals: Attraction and retention of professional nurses. *Nursing Administration Quarterly, 26*(1), 45–54. https://doi.org/10.1097/00006216-200201000-00006.

McGillis Hall, L., Doran, D., & Pink, L. (2007). Impact of work environments on nurses' health and performance. *Nursing Leadership, 20*(3), 12–20. https://doi.org/10.12927/cjnl.2007.19165.

McVicar, A. (2003). Workplace stress in nursing: A literature review. *Journal of Advanced Nursing, 44*(6), 633–642. https://doi.org/10.1046/j.0309-2402.2003.02853.x.

Melchior, F. (2004). Feminist approaches to nursing history. *Western Journal of Nursing Research, 26*(3), 340–355.

Melnyk, B. M., Fineout-Overholt, E., Stillwell, S. B., & Williamson, K. M. (2014). Evidence-based practice: Step by step: The seven steps of evidence-based practice. *American Journal of Nursing, 110*(1), 51–53. https://doi.org/10.1097/01.NAJ.0000366056.06605.d2.

NHS England. (2018–2019). NHS England funding and resource 2018–19: Supporting next steps for the NHS Five Year Forward View. https://www.england.nhs.uk/publication/nhs-england-funding-and-resource-2018-19-supporting-next-steps-for-the-nhs-five-year-forward-view/

Pfettscher, S. A. (2021). Florence Nightingale: Modern nursing. In M. R. Alligood (Ed.), *Nursing theorists and their work*, 52–70.

Pulido-Martos, M., Augusto-Landa, J. M., & Lopez-Zafra, E. (2012). Sources of stress in nursing students: A systematic review of quantitative studies. *International Nursing Review, 59*(1), 15–25. https://doi.org/10.1111/j.1466-7657.2011.00939.x.

Rafferty, A. M. (1996). *The politics of nursing knowledge*. Routledge.

Roberts, S. J. (2016). Oppressed group behavior: Implications for nursing. *Advances in Nursing Science, 39*(3), 213–223. https://doi.org/10.1097/ANS.0000000000000121.

Rudman, A., & Gustavsson, J. P. (2012). Burnout during nursing education predicts lower occupational preparedness and future clinical performance: A longitudinal study. *International Journal of Nursing Studies, 49*(8), 988–1001. https://doi.org/10.1016/j.ijnurstu.2012.03.010.

Schaufeli, W. B. (2017). Burnout: A short socio-cultural history. In , *Burnout, fatigue, exhaustion: An interdisciplinary perspective on a modern affliction*, 105–127.

Shanafelt, T. D., Ripp, J., & Trockel, M. (2020). Understanding and addressing sources of anxiety among healthcare professionals during the COVID-19 pandemic. *JAMA, 323*(21), 2133–2134. https://doi.org/10.1001/jama.2020.5893.

Shaw, L., Masood, M., Neufeld, K., Connelly, D. M., Stanley, M., Guitar, N. A., … Nikkhou, A. (2024). A conceptual framework for defining work disparities: A case of nurses in long-term care. *WORK*.

Sitzman, K., & Ely, D. (2010). *Mentoring new nurses: An essential guide for professional development*. Springer Publishing Company.

Stokes, J. (1999). Health care reform in the 1980s and 1990s: The effect on nurses. *Nursing Economics, 17*(1), 44–49.

Stone, R. I. (2001). The impact of hospital mergers on nursing: A review of the literature. *Journal of Healthcare Management, 46*(5), 356–366.

UK Central Council for Nursing, Midwifery and Health Visiting. (1986). *Project 2000: A new preparation for practice*. UKCC.

UK Central Council for Nursing, Midwifery and Health Visiting. (1999). *Fitness for practice: The UKCC Commission for Nursing and Midwifery Education*. UKCC.

Watson, R. (1995). Education and training of enrolled nurses: Lessons from history. *Nurse Education Today, 15*(2), 108–113. https://doi.org/10.1016/S0260-6917(95)80106-7.

CHAPTER 2

What Is Attrition in Higher Education?

Amanda Costello

Introduction

Attrition in higher education refers to the phenomenon of students leaving their academic programmes before completion, a challenge that has widespread consequences for students, educational institutions, and society at large. The issue is of significant concern because it not only reflects the failure to complete academic goals but also has broader implications for the quality and accessibility of higher education. As Tinto (1993, p. 95) suggests, student attrition 'represents the culmination of a variety of factors, often linked to students' sense of belonging and engagement within the academic environment.' High attrition rates can negatively impact institutional reputation, reducing the perceived value of a degree and diminishing the university's role in fostering educated professionals. Furthermore, the economic consequences of attrition are considerable, as the loss of students results in financial strain for educational institutions while reducing the pool of skilled graduates entering the workforce. The broader societal implications include hindered economic growth and a reduction in social mobility, particularly among students from underrepresented backgrounds.

The causes of attrition in higher education are multilayered, often influenced by a combination of academic, financial, psychological, and institutional factors. These challenges can be categorised into academic preparedness, financial constraints, psychological well-being, and institutional support. A lack of academic readiness or struggling with coursework, for example, is often linked to high dropout rates, especially in rigorous programmes. Financial difficulties are another significant barrier, with students from low-income backgrounds facing increased risks of leaving their studies due to the pressures of tuition fees, living costs, and the need to balance work and study (Tinto, 2012). Psychological factors such as stress, mental health issues, and a lack of social integration further contribute to attrition. As Pascarella and Terenzini (2005, p. 276) argue, 'students who feel disconnected or unsupported by their peers or faculty are more likely to withdraw from their studies, as they lack the emotional and social resources to cope with academic challenges.' Institutional factors, such as inadequate advising, limited financial aid, or a lack of student-centred support services, also play a critical role in influencing retention.

Understanding and addressing student attrition is essential for improving retention rates, which are increasingly seen as a measure of institutional effectiveness. By addressing the underlying causes of attrition, educational institutions can enhance student experience, increase graduation rates, and succeed in their mission of producing well-prepared professionals. Effective strategies include improving student engagement through active learning, offering financial support and academic advising, fostering a sense of belonging, and implementing early intervention programmes (Kuh et al., 2007). By addressing the complex, interrelated factors that contribute to attrition, higher education institutions can create an environment where students are more likely to persist and complete their academic journeys.

This chapter critically examines the concept of attrition in higher education, discussing key themes such as student engagement, financial constraints, academic preparedness, institutional support, and sociodemographic influences. By exploring the interplay of these factors, we aim to provide a comprehensive understanding of student attrition and offer insights into strategies for improving retention rates in higher education.

Key Themes in Attrition in Higher Education

STUDENT ENGAGEMENT AND MOTIVATION

Student engagement is a crucial determinant of retention in higher education. Lack of engagement can result from various factors, including uninteresting coursework, lack of peer interaction, and ineffective teaching methods (Kuh et al., 2007). Motivation plays a critical role; students with intrinsic motivation are more likely to overcome challenges and persist, whereas those with extrinsic motivation may struggle when faced with difficulties (Deci & Ryan, 1985).

Student Engagement as a Determinant of Retention in Higher Education: The Case of Undergraduate Nursing Students

Student engagement is widely regarded as one of the most significant factors influencing retention in undergraduate nursing students. According to Tinto (1993), students who actively participate in both academic and extracurricular activities demonstrate higher levels of persistence, which ultimately leads to improved retention rates. Tinto argues that engagement helps students to form connections within the academic community, which in turn enhances their commitment to completing their programmes. Engagement promotes a sense of belonging, motivation, and academic commitment, all of which are essential for students to continue and successfully complete their studies. In professional programmes such as nursing, where students must navigate both theoretical coursework and demanding clinical placements, engagement is particularly crucial in ensuring retention and progression. As explained by Shaw (2018, p. 47), 'nursing students who feel connected to their program and peers are more likely to remain in the program and ultimately graduate.'

Engagement in higher education can take multiple forms, including behavioural, emotional, and cognitive engagement. Behavioural engagement refers to active participation in classroom activities, attending lectures, and involvement in student organisations or campus events (Fredricks et al., 2004). Research by Kuh (2009) supports the idea that behavioural engagement, such as attending class and participating in co-curricular activities, is strongly correlated with academic success and retention. Emotional engagement involves developing a sense of connection with peers, faculty, and the institution itself, which enhances students' feelings of belonging and satisfaction (Fredricks et al., 2004). Emotional engagement is critical for students to feel integrated within the academic community, which in turn encourages them to persist in their studies. Cognitive engagement, however, relates to the depth of intellectual investment in learning, such as critical thinking, problem-solving, and self-directed learning. As Fredricks et al. (2004) explain, cognitive engagement requires students to approach learning with a sense of responsibility and curiosity, which stimulates a deeper understanding and academic achievement. The interchange between these types of engagement significantly impacts students' academic success and their likelihood of persisting in their programmes. As summarised by Astin (1984, p. 297), 'student involvement is a key to academic success and retention,' emphasising the importance of holistic engagement in shaping students' educational experiences.

Engagement Challenges in Undergraduate Nursing Education

Retention in undergraduate nursing programmes presents a unique set of challenges. Nursing students often experience high levels of stress due to the rigorous academic and clinical demands of their education (Crombie et al., 2013). As Crombie et al. (2013, p. 170) consider, 'nursing students experience a higher level of stress compared to students in other disciplines, largely due to the dual demands of academic and clinical responsibilities.' Unlike other undergraduate disciplines, nursing students must balance theoretical learning with practical placements in healthcare settings, which can be physically and emotionally exhausting. A lack of engagement due to academic struggles, social isolation, or overwhelming clinical expectations can contribute to higher attrition rates in nursing programmes compared to other disciplines (Glossop, 2002). According to Glossop (2002, p. 116), 'the unique challenges faced by nursing students, such as the stress of clinical placements and the pressure to perform academically, often lead to higher dropout rates in nursing programs.'

A key factor contributing to disengagement in nursing education is the nature of coursework and clinical experiences. Nursing curricula are often content heavy, requiring students to master complex theoretical concepts alongside developing hands-on clinical competencies. As described by Eick et al. (2012, p. 282), 'students frequently struggle with the volume and complexity of the coursework, which can undermine their confidence and academic motivation.' If students find the material uninteresting or excessively difficult without adequate support, their engagement can decrease. Additionally, clinical placements can be a source of both engagement and disengagement. Positive clinical experiences, where students feel supported by mentors and integrated into the healthcare team, enhance engagement and motivation. Eick et al. (2012, p. 283) emphasise that 'supportive clinical placements where students feel part of the healthcare team have been shown to improve retention, as they foster a sense of professional identity and engagement.' However, negative experiences, such as unsupportive clinical environments, high-pressure workloads, or lack of preparedness, can lead to stress, burnout, and disengagement, ultimately increasing the likelihood of attrition (Eick et al., 2012).

Another significant challenge in nursing retention is peer interaction and social support. Nursing students often work in small cohorts, which can provide a strong sense of community and shared experience. However, if students struggle to build peer relationships or feel isolated, disengagement can occur. As Astin (1999, p. 253) argues, 'students who develop strong social connections and engage with their peers are more likely to remain in their academic programs, as they experience a greater sense of belonging and support.' Research suggests that students who form social connections within their academic environment are more likely to persist (Astin, 1999). Supportive peer relationships contribute to academic encouragement, knowledge sharing, and emotional support, all of which mitigate the risk of dropout. Nursing students in particular benefit from peer mentorship programmes and study groups, which help them to navigate the demanding nature of their studies. As illuminated by McDonald et al. (2016, p. 89), 'peer mentorship programs have proven to be effective in providing students with both academic guidance and emotional support, fostering a more engaged and resilient student body.'

The Role of Teaching Methods and Institutional Support

Effective pedagogy plays a crucial role in stimulating engagement in nursing education. Traditional lecture-based approaches, which rely heavily on passive learning, can contribute to disengagement if students do not feel actively involved in the learning process. According to Kuh et al. (2008, p. 151), 'passive learning environments that do not engage students actively in the learning process have been linked to lower levels of academic achievement and engagement.' When students are not given opportunities to actively participate, they may struggle to see the relevance of the material, leading to a lack of motivation and reduced persistence. In contrast, active learning strategies such as simulation-based learning, case-based discussions, and problem-based learning enhance engagement by providing hands-on, real-world applications of theoretical knowledge. Kuh et al. (2008, p. 153) further argue that 'active learning strategies promote deeper understanding and help students connect theoretical concepts with practical experiences, which is essential in nursing education.' These strategies allow nursing students to engage in authentic problem-solving and critical thinking—skills that are vital for clinical practice.

Simulation training in particular has been shown to increase nursing students' confidence, clinical competence, and overall engagement in their studies. As Cant and Cooper (2010, p. 285) suggest, 'simulation allows students to experience realistic clinical scenarios in a controlled environment, providing them with the opportunity to practice and refine their clinical skills without the risk of patient harm.' This hands-on approach enables students to better retain knowledge and develop practical skills that they will use in real-life clinical settings. Furthermore, simulation training has been found to improve students' decision-making abilities, critical thinking, and ability to manage complex clinical situations (Cant & Cooper, 2010). This increased competence not only boosts students' confidence but also contributes to their overall engagement with the nursing programme, as they feel more prepared and capable in their learning journey.

Institutional support also plays a vital role in nursing student retention. Universities that offer mentorship programmes, academic advising, and mental health support services create an environment where students feel valued and supported. According to Jeffreys (2007, p. 37), 'institutional support systems, including academic advising and mentorship, are crucial in helping students navigate the academic and emotional challenges they face during their nursing education.' Such support systems ensure that students have access to resources that help them to succeed academically and manage stress. Jeffreys (2007, p. 39) emphasises that 'early identification of at-risk students and providing timely academic support are essential strategies in improving retention rates.' By intervening early, nursing programmes can provide students with the additional resources and guidance they need to overcome challenges before they become insurmountable, ultimately leading to improved retention.

Additionally, fostering strong faculty–student relationships through accessible and supportive educators can significantly enhance student engagement and motivation. Research indicates that 'students who perceive their faculty as approachable and supportive are more likely to feel connected to the program and motivated to persist' (Bastable, 2008, p. 221). Faculty members who take the time to engage with students, offer guidance, and provide timely feedback create an atmosphere of trust and respect, which is essential for student retention and success. Bastable (2008, p. 223) argues, 'faculty who serve as mentors and provide individualised support contribute to a learning environment where students feel valued, ultimately promoting their academic success and overall engagement in the program.' This type of relationship can serve as a protective factor against attrition by nurturing a sense of belonging and support, both academically and emotionally.

The Impact of Motivation on Nursing Student Retention

Motivation plays a crucial role in determining the level of student engagement and, consequently, retention. According to the self-determination theory of Deci and Ryan (1985), motivation can be categorised into intrinsic and extrinsic forms. Intrinsic motivation, which arises from personal interest and enjoyment of learning, is a powerful driver of persistence. Deci and Ryan (1985, p. 35) explain that 'intrinsic motivation refers to doing something because it is inherently interesting or enjoyable, rather than for some separable consequence.' Nursing students who are intrinsically motivated, often driven by a strong desire to help others and make a meaningful difference in healthcare, are more likely to engage deeply with their coursework. These students are not merely focused on external rewards such as grades or career prospects, but are motivated by a sense of purpose and a genuine passion for nursing. As Luthans and Youssef (2007, p. 145) suggest, 'students who are intrinsically motivated often exhibit higher levels of persistence and engage in deeper learning, as they are driven by personal values and the internal satisfaction derived from mastering content.'

For example, nursing students who are passionate about patient care often go above and beyond in their studies, seeking out additional learning opportunities, engaging with faculty, and demonstrating a high level of commitment to their clinical placements. According to Sinclair et al. (2015, p. 78), 'nursing students who identify with the values of the profession, such as empathy and altruism, often show greater resilience in the face of academic and clinical challenges.' These students tend to persist through difficulties because their motivation is seated in a sense of personal satisfaction rather than external validation.

Conversely, extrinsic motivation, which is driven by external rewards such as grades, job prospects, or financial incentives, can be less sustainable. Deci and Ryan (1985, p. 36) describe extrinsic motivation as 'doing something for the sake of achieving some separable outcome, such as obtaining a reward or avoiding punishment.' Nursing students who enter the programme primarily due to external pressures such as the desire for job security, family expectations, or financial rewards may initially engage with their studies but are at greater risk of disengagement when faced with the demanding nature of nursing education. These students may prioritise grades over a deep understanding of the material, and when they encounter academic or clinical difficulties, they may struggle to maintain motivation. According to Ryan and Deci (2000, p. 61), 'students motivated by external factors often experience lower levels of satisfaction and well-being, which can lead to reduced persistence and a higher likelihood of attrition.'

An example of extrinsic motivation in nursing education can be seen in students who focus solely on achieving high grades or securing a well-paying job after graduation. These students may lose sight of the deeper purpose of nursing, such as patient care and making a positive impact on healthcare, which can lead to burnout or disengagement when the workload becomes overwhelming. As Jones and Watt (2011, p. 24) note, 'students who focus on external rewards such as grades and job prospects may find it difficult to stay motivated when faced with the emotionally demanding and rigorous nature of nursing education.'

This highlights the importance of harnessing intrinsic motivation through meaningful learning experiences, supportive faculty interactions, and opportunities for professional identity development. As Schunk et al. (2008, p. 255) suggest, 'intrinsic motivation can be nurtured by creating learning environments that are relevant, challenging, and aligned with students' personal interests and values.' In nursing education this can be achieved by designing curricula that emphasise the real-world application of theoretical knowledge, providing opportunities for students to engage in clinical practice, and encouraging students to reflect on the broader impact of their work on patient care. Furthermore, supportive faculty interactions can strengthen intrinsic motivation by helping students to connect their learning to their personal values and career goals. As DeWitt and Carr (2015, p. 42) point out, 'faculty who foster a sense of belonging and purpose in students are instrumental in helping them navigate the emotional and academic challenges of nursing education, promoting long-term motivation and retention.'

Overall, while extrinsic motivation can serve as an initial driver for nursing students, intrinsic motivation plays a more sustainable and meaningful role in stimulating deep engagement, persistence, and retention in nursing programmes. By cultivating intrinsic motivation through a combination of personal interest, purpose-driven learning experiences, and faculty support, nursing programmes can help students not only to succeed academically but also to develop into compassionate, resilient healthcare professionals.

Strategies for Enhancing Nursing Student Engagement and Retention

Given the critical role of engagement in nursing student retention, institutions can implement several strategies to improve persistence rates:

- *Creating Supportive Learning Environments*: Ensuring that nursing students have access to academic support services, counselling, and mentorship programmes can help them to manage the challenges of their education.
- *Enhancing Clinical Experiences*: Partnering with healthcare organisations to provide high-quality, supportive clinical placements can improve students' engagement and sense of professional identity.
- *Promoting Peer Support Networks*: Encouraging study groups, peer mentoring, and cohort-building activities can foster a sense of community and shared purpose.
- *Utilising Active Learning Strategies*: Incorporating simulation training, case-based learning, and problem-solving exercises can make coursework more engaging and relevant.
- *Faculty Development and Support*: Training educators in student-centred teaching approaches and mentorship techniques can improve faculty–student interactions and overall student engagement.

Student engagement is a multilayered and critical determinant of retention in higher education, particularly in demanding fields such as nursing. As Tinto (1993, p. 96) explains, 'students who are actively engaged in the learning process are more likely to persist and succeed in their studies.' Engagement in higher education is not a singular experience but involves multiple dimensions – academic, social, and emotional – that contribute to a student's sense of belonging, motivation, and commitment. In the context of nursing education, where students are required to navigate both theoretical coursework and rigorous clinical placements, engagement becomes even more vital. According to Kuh et al. (2008, p. 7), 'student engagement, defined as the time and energy students invest in educationally purposeful activities, has been consistently linked to positive outcomes, including retention and academic success.' Ensuring that undergraduate nursing students are actively involved in both academic and clinical aspects of their education requires a concerted effort from educators, administrators, and students themselves.

A key factor in fostering engagement is addressing the elements that contribute to disengagement. Nursing education presents unique challenges, such as demanding coursework that requires mastery of both theoretical and practical knowledge. If students find the material overwhelming or disengaging, they may begin to disengage, leading to lower retention rates. As Lockhart and DeLuca (2019, p. 35) note, 'students who experience academic struggles, particularly in high-stakes fields such as nursing, may feel alienated and isolated, which can negatively impact their motivation to persist.' In addition to academic difficulties, unsupportive clinical placements are a significant contributor to disengagement. Nursing students often face challenging clinical environments where they are expected to apply their theoretical knowledge in real-world settings. A lack of support from clinical mentors or staff can leave students feeling inadequate and unsupported, ultimately contributing to burnout and attrition. According to Eick et al. (2012, p. 293), 'negative clinical experiences, such as feeling unsupported or overburdened, can cause nursing students to question their career choice and reduce their engagement with the program.'

Furthermore, a lack of peer interaction and social support can exacerbate feelings of isolation and contribute to disengagement. In nursing education, students often work in small cohorts, and the strength of peer relationships can play a significant role in retention. Research by Astin (1999, p. 28) highlights that 'students who have strong connections with their peers are more likely to persist in their studies because they feel a sense of community and support.' This sense of belonging is crucial in a demanding field like nursing, where students are often required to cope with high levels of stress and emotional intensity. Without the emotional and social support of peers, students may struggle to cope with the challenges of nursing education, leading to a higher likelihood of attrition.

To address these factors, institutions must foster an environment that supports intrinsic motivation and meaningful participation. Intrinsic motivation, defined by Deci and Ryan (1985) as the drive to engage in an activity for its inherent satisfaction, plays a crucial role in nursing students' persistence. When students are intrinsically motivated by a desire to care for others and make a difference in the healthcare system, they are more likely to engage deeply in both their academic and clinical work. As Cant and Cooper (2010, p. 286) argue, 'nursing students who are intrinsically motivated are more likely to demonstrate resilience, persistence, and a high level of engagement in their studies.' Institutions can foster intrinsic motivation by designing curricula that emphasise the real-world impact of nursing and by creating learning environments that value the personal and emotional growth of students.

In addition, enabling an inclusive and supportive institutional culture is essential for improving engagement. This includes providing mentorship programmes, academic advising, and peer support systems that create a sense of community and help students to navigate the emotional and academic challenges of nursing education. According to Jeffreys (2007, p. 62), 'mentorship and support systems play a critical role in helping nursing students feel valued and connected to their program, which can significantly improve retention rates.' By creating spaces where students can build relationships with faculty, peers, and mentors, institutions can reduce feelings of isolation and increase engagement.

Given the ongoing global shortage of nurses, improving engagement and retention in nursing education is not only beneficial for students but also essential for the future of healthcare. The nursing profession is critical to the delivery of healthcare services worldwide, and ensuring that students successfully complete their education is crucial for addressing staffing shortages and improving patient outcomes. As Benner et al. (2010, p. 29) emphasise, 'retaining nursing students through supportive educational practices is essential for ensuring a well-prepared workforce that can meet the growing demands of healthcare.' Ultimately, fostering student engagement in nursing education benefits not only individual students but also the healthcare system as a whole, helping to ensure that future nurses are equipped to meet the challenges of the profession.

FINANCIAL CONSTRAINTS

Financial barriers are one of the most cited reasons for student attrition. Rising tuition fees, the burden of student loans, and the need to balance work and study create immense pressure on students (Hossler et al., 2009a). Low-income students are at a particularly high risk of dropping out due to their inability to afford educational expenses. Financial aid programmes and scholarships play a vital role in mitigating this issue; however, gaps in funding still exist, leading to financial stress that impacts student retention (Goldrick-Rab, 2016).

Financial Barriers to Retention in Undergraduate Nursing Programmes

Financial barriers are one of the most significant challenges contributing to student attrition, particularly for undergraduate nursing students. Rising tuition fees, the burden of student loans, and the need to balance work and study create immense pressure on students pursuing higher education. This pressure is even more pronounced in nursing programmes, where the academic workload is intense and clinical placements require substantial time and commitment outside the classroom. As a result, students in nursing programmes face unique financial challenges that can directly affect their retention and progression.

For many nursing students, the financial strain of tuition fees and living costs can become overwhelming. Rising tuition fees and associated costs, such as textbooks, uniforms, and clinical placements, have made it increasingly difficult for students from low-income backgrounds to persist in their studies (Hossler et al., 2009b). The financial burden is particularly severe for students who need to work part time or full time to support themselves, as this can lead to physical and mental exhaustion, further impeding academic performance. Consequently, low-income nursing students are at an elevated risk of dropping out due to their inability to afford the necessary educational expenses.

Financial aid programmes such as scholarships, grants, and student loans play a crucial role in helping nursing students to manage these costs. However, despite the availability of financial assistance, significant gaps in funding still exist. These gaps often leave students in precarious financial situations, making it difficult for them to meet their educational and living expenses without taking on significant debt (Goldrick-Rab, 2016). The lack of sufficient financial support not only adds stress but also affects the students' overall well-being, which can lead to disengagement and reduced motivation to persist in the nursing programme.

Moreover, the financial pressures experienced by nursing students can affect their emotional and cognitive engagement. Students who are focused on securing financial resources may struggle to invest fully in their academic studies or clinical experiences, impacting both their academic success and the development of critical skills necessary for effective nursing practice. Therefore, institutions need to recognise the impact of financial stress on nursing students' retention and provide additional support, such as targeted financial aid initiatives and flexible work-study programmes, to help alleviate these barriers.

By addressing the financial challenges faced by nursing students, educational institutions can help to reduce attrition rates and improve retention within nursing programmes. Efforts to enhance financial aid offerings and create more affordable educational opportunities can support students in balancing the financial pressures of higher education with the rigorous demands of nursing coursework and clinical placements.

ACADEMIC PREPAREDNESS AND PERFORMANCE

Many students enter higher education without the necessary academic skills to succeed. Poor academic preparation in secondary education, especially in subjects like mathematics and writing, can lead to difficulties in coping with university-level coursework (Bailey et al., 2010). Students who struggle academically often experience lower self-esteem and increased stress, which can contribute to their decision to leave. Effective remedial programmes, tutoring services, and mentorship initiatives have been shown to enhance student performance and reduce attrition rates (Tinto, 2012).

Academic Barriers to Retention in Undergraduate Nursing Programmes

Many students entering higher education, including those in undergraduate nursing programmes, face significant academic challenges due to insufficient preparation in secondary education. Students who have not developed strong foundational skills in key areas such as mathematics, writing, and critical thinking often struggle to keep up with the rigorous academic demands of university-level coursework (Bailey et al., 2010). For nursing students, these challenges can be especially pronounced, as they are required to master complex theoretical concepts in subjects like anatomy, pharmacology, and nursing theory, all of which demand a solid understanding of mathematics and writing.

The gap in academic preparation can create significant hurdles for nursing students, leading to feelings of inadequacy, frustration, and lower self-esteem. These emotional responses, coupled with the academic pressures of nursing coursework, often result in heightened stress, which further impedes their ability to engage with the material and succeed in their studies. For nursing students, the inability to manage academic demands, particularly in foundational subjects, can contribute to disengagement, decreased motivation, and, ultimately, higher attrition rates.

In addition to academic challenges, nursing students must also contend with the practical, hands-on aspects of their education, which require a different set of skills. If students are not academically prepared for the theoretical component, they may also struggle to perform well during clinical placements, where they are expected to apply their learning in real-world healthcare settings. This dual challenge of theoretical and clinical demands makes the need for strong academic skills even more critical in ensuring nursing students' success and retention.

Effective remedial programmes and academic support services are essential in addressing these barriers. For nursing students, tutoring services, writing assistance, and mathematics support can significantly improve academic performance. Additionally, mentorship initiatives that pair students with experienced faculty or senior nursing students can provide valuable guidance and encouragement. These initiatives help to bridge the gap between the students' current academic skills and the expectations of the nursing programme, offering personalised assistance to help them build the necessary competencies (Tinto, 2012).

Research has shown that institutions that implement targeted academic support for students struggling with foundational skills see improvements in student retention and academic performance. For nursing students in particular, early identification of academic struggles, followed by timely intervention, is crucial. Programmes that offer individualised academic support, workshops focused on study strategies, and peer mentoring not only improve students' academic abilities but also foster a sense of belonging and support, which is key to retention.

By recognising the academic challenges faced by nursing students and providing the appropriate resources, higher education institutions can reduce attrition rates and promote academic success. Tailored academic support programmes that address the unique needs of nursing students can help to ensure that these future healthcare professionals are prepared to meet the demands of their coursework and clinical placements, leading to increased persistence and success in their nursing programmes.

INSTITUTIONAL SUPPORT AND STUDENT SERVICES

The level of institutional support plays a significant role in student retention. Institutions that offer comprehensive academic advising, mental health counselling, career services, and mentorship programmes tend to have lower attrition rates (Seidman, 2005). First-year experience programmes, which include orientation and academic skill-building sessions, are particularly effective in improving student integration into the university environment (Pascarella & Terenzini, 2005). Additionally, faculty involvement in student success, including personalised support and active engagement in student development, can foster a sense of belonging and encourage persistence.

The Role of Institutional Support in Retention of Undergraduate Nursing Students

The level of institutional support is a critical factor in promoting retention, particularly for undergraduate nursing students, who face unique challenges in balancing rigorous academic coursework with demanding clinical placements. Institutions that provide comprehensive academic advising, mental health counselling, career services, and mentorship programmes are better equipped to address the holistic needs of their nursing students, which in turn contributes to lower attrition rates (Seidman, 2005). These support services are essential in helping students to navigate both the academic and emotional challenges they encounter throughout their nursing education.

For nursing students, academic advising is particularly important, as it ensures that students are on track with course requirements and that they are aware of opportunities for support when academic struggles arise. Nursing programmes often have complex curricula with sequential course requirements, and students need personalised guidance to ensure that they stay on track, avoid burnout, and manage the demands of both theory and clinical practice. Comprehensive advising services can also help students to make informed decisions about their career paths and academic goals, thus enhancing their motivation to persist in the programme.

Mental health support is another crucial area for nursing students, who frequently experience high levels of stress due to the challenging nature of their studies and the emotional demands of clinical placements. Mental health counselling services can provide nursing students with a space to manage stress, address feelings of anxiety, and work through the emotional complexities that arise in both the classroom and clinical settings. Institutions that prioritise mental health services contribute to the overall well-being of their students, which directly impacts their ability to engage in their studies and complete their programmes.

First-year experience programmes are also beneficial for undergraduate nursing students, particularly those entering the programme with little understanding of the expectations and demands of the profession. These programmes, which include orientation sessions and academic skill-building workshops, help students to transition smoothly into university life and develop the skills needed to succeed in their nursing studies. For nursing students, these programmes can include specialised sessions on study techniques for nursing courses, time management strategies for balancing clinical placements, and information on available support services. These programmes help nursing students to feel more integrated into the university environment, which is vital for fostering a sense of belonging and community within the nursing cohort (Pascarella & Terenzini, 2005).

In addition to institutional services, faculty involvement plays a significant role in student success and retention. In nursing education, faculty engagement in student development such as providing personalised support, fostering active learning environments, and offering mentorship opportunities can greatly enhance students' sense of belonging and academic persistence. Nursing faculty who actively engage with students, both in and outside the classroom, can help students to navigate the challenges of their education and provide the encouragement needed to persevere through difficult coursework and clinical experiences. Faculty mentorship helps to create a supportive environment where students feel that their personal and academic struggles are acknowledged and addressed, which is crucial for improving retention rates in nursing programmes.

When nursing students feel supported by both their peers and faculty members, they are more likely to persist in their programmes, perform better academically, and develop a stronger professional identity. Thus comprehensive institutional support, tailored to the unique needs of nursing students, is essential in fostering student success and ensuring the retention of future healthcare professionals.

SOCIODEMOGRAPHIC INFLUENCES

Demographic factors such as age, gender, ethnicity, and socioeconomic background significantly impact attrition rates. First-generation college students, racial minorities, and nontraditional students (e.g., adult learners) face unique challenges that affect their ability to complete their studies (Swail et al., 2003). These challenges include lack of family support, cultural barriers, and work–family balance issues. Universities that implement targeted support programmes for underrepresented groups often see improvements in retention rates (Engle & Tinto, 2008).

Demographic Factors Influencing Attrition in Undergraduate Nursing Programmes

Demographic factors such as age, gender, ethnicity, and socioeconomic background significantly influence attrition rates among students in higher education, and these factors are particularly impactful for undergraduate nursing students. Nursing programmes often attract a diverse student body, with students from a variety of age groups, cultural backgrounds, and socioeconomic statuses. As such, nursing students from underrepresented and nontraditional backgrounds may face unique challenges that affect their ability to persist and complete their studies.

First-generation college students, those whose parents did not attend college, often face additional obstacles in navigating the academic landscape of higher education. Many first-generation nursing students lack the familial knowledge of how to succeed in a rigorous academic environment, which can lead to difficulties in academic planning, securing financial aid, and balancing academic responsibilities with family obligations. These challenges can be especially pronounced in nursing programmes, where students are expected to meet high academic standards while also completing demanding clinical placements.

Similarly, racial minorities in nursing programmes may experience cultural barriers that hinder their academic success and social integration. These barriers can manifest as feelings of isolation, discrimination, or a lack of cultural representation in faculty and clinical staff. Racially diverse nursing students may also face societal biases that affect their confidence and sense of belonging, leading to disengagement and increased attrition (Swail et al., 2003). Given the importance of cultural competence in nursing, these students can feel excluded from educational spaces that do not reflect or respect their experiences, which can negatively impact their retention.

Nontraditional students, such as adult learners, also face unique challenges in nursing education. Adult learners often return to school after a significant gap, balancing educational demands with work, family, and other life responsibilities. The need to juggle multiple roles can lead to high levels of stress and burnout. In nursing programmes, where clinical hours and exams require extensive time commitments, nontraditional students may struggle to maintain the balance needed to succeed academically. Additionally, the lack of peer relationships and social integration can create feelings of isolation, further contributing to attrition.

Socioeconomic background also plays a pivotal role in the retention of nursing students. Students from low-income backgrounds may experience additional barriers, such as limited access to necessary resources like textbooks, clinical uniforms, or transportation to clinical placements. They are more likely to work part-time or full-time jobs to support themselves, which can lead to exhaustion and a decrease in their ability to focus on their academic and clinical responsibilities. The financial burden of nursing education combined with the costs of clinical placements and licensure exams can also discourage retention in the programme.

To mitigate these demographic challenges, universities that implement targeted support programmes for underrepresented groups, including mentorship programmes, financial aid, and tailored academic resources, have seen improvements in retention rates (Engle & Tinto, 2008). These programmes are particularly beneficial in nursing programmes, where students from diverse backgrounds can greatly benefit from a supportive, inclusive learning environment that acknowledges and addresses their unique needs.

Strategies to Reduce Attrition in Undergraduate Nursing Programmes

To address attrition in undergraduate nursing programmes, higher education institutions must adopt a multifaceted approach that not only tackles the academic and social challenges but also addresses the financial and emotional factors that contribute to student disengagement. Key strategies are presented next.

ENHANCING STUDENT ENGAGEMENT

Creating interactive learning environments that actively engage students in the learning process is essential for reducing attrition. In nursing education, this can be achieved by promoting collaborative projects, case studies, and hands-on simulation experiences that mirror real-world healthcare settings. Student–faculty interactions are also critical in fostering engagement, as faculty members who are invested in student success and development can create a sense of connection and support. For nursing students, who often face academic and clinical challenges, regular interactions with faculty can increase motivation and encourage persistence through difficulties.

PROVIDING FINANCIAL ASSISTANCE

Given the high cost of nursing education, providing financial assistance is crucial to ensure that students are not forced to abandon their studies due to financial strain. This can include expanding scholarship opportunities, implementing flexible payment plans, and increasing awareness of financial aid options for students. Nursing students from low-income backgrounds may also benefit from emergency funding programmes that can help to cover unexpected expenses, such as the costs associated with clinical placements or licensure exams.

IMPROVING ACADEMIC PREPAREDNESS

One of the key factors contributing to attrition is academic preparedness. Many nursing students struggle with the demanding curriculum, particularly in subjects that require strong foundational skills in mathematics, science, and writing. Institutions can improve high school-to-college transition programmes that provide academic support and readiness training for nursing students. Offering preparatory courses for subjects like anatomy, chemistry, and statistics can give students the tools they need to succeed. Additionally, integrating learning support services such as tutoring and writing centres into nursing programmes can provide students with ongoing assistance throughout their studies.

STRENGTHENING INSTITUTIONAL SUPPORT

Institutional support is vital in ensuring the retention of nursing students, particularly for those from underrepresented backgrounds. Universities should invest in developing comprehensive advising systems that provide academic and career counselling, especially for students who may not have the familial support to navigate higher education. Expanding mental health resources is equally crucial, as nursing students often experience high levels of stress due to the academic and emotional demands of their programme. Increased access to counselling services can help students to cope with stress, anxiety, and burnout. Additionally, career development services can guide nursing students in exploring job opportunities after graduation, which can help to maintain their motivation to persist in the programme.

SUPPORTING DIVERSE STUDENT POPULATIONS

Nursing programmes must implement mentorship programmes specifically for first-generation students and students from underrepresented backgrounds. These programmes pair students with faculty, senior students, or healthcare professionals who can provide guidance, support, and career insights. Moreover, childcare services for student-parents and promoting inclusivity on campus can address the specific challenges faced by these populations. Creating a culture of inclusivity, where all students regardless of their age, gender, ethnicity, or socioeconomic status feel valued and supported, is key to reducing attrition and ensuring that nursing students successfully complete their programmes.

These strategies, when implemented comprehensively, can help institutions to address the complex challenges faced by undergraduate nursing students and reduce attrition rates. Tailoring support to the unique needs of nursing students while also focusing on broader institutional strategies to improve retention can ensure that nursing students from diverse backgrounds not only complete their programmes but thrive in their professional journeys.

Conclusion

Attrition in higher education is a multilayered challenge shaped by a variety of interconnected factors that extend beyond academic performance. These factors include, but are not limited to, student engagement, financial constraints, academic preparedness, institutional support, and sociodemographic influences. Student engagement plays a crucial role in retention, as students who feel connected to their peers, professors, and academic content are more likely to persist in their studies. Financial constraints, including the rising costs of tuition, textbooks, and living expenses, can lead to students discontinuing their education due to the burden of debt or lack of sufficient resources. Additionally, academic preparedness is a major determinant, as students who enter higher education without the necessary foundational knowledge or skills may struggle to succeed, leading to a higher likelihood of dropout.

Institutional support, or the lack thereof, significantly affects student retention. Adequate advising, counselling services, mental health resources, and academic tutoring can make a difference in a student's ability to overcome personal and academic challenges. Moreover, institutions that offer flexible learning environments, including online or hybrid models, may be better equipped to accommodate students with diverse needs and schedules. Sociodemographic factors such as race, gender, socioeconomic background, and family responsibilities also play a pivotal role in attrition rates, as certain groups may face additional barriers that hinder their ability to succeed in higher education.

Addressing attrition therefore requires a holistic approach that involves collaboration among educators, administrators, policymakers, and students themselves. It is essential that institutions create a culture of inclusivity and support that empowers students to overcome challenges and persist toward graduation. Educators must be trained to recognize early warning signs of disengagement or academic struggle and respond with tailored interventions. Administrators should focus on creating policies that reduce financial burdens, such as scholarships, work-study opportunities, or affordable housing options. Policymakers must advocate for funding initiatives that make higher education more accessible, especially for underrepresented and disadvantaged populations.

Furthermore, students themselves must be proactive in seeking support when needed and engaging with the resources available to them. By promoting a sense of community, belonging, and ownership in the learning process, institutions can build an environment where students feel motivated to persist. Implementing targeted interventions that address specific causes of attrition, such as academic remediation for underprepared students or financial literacy workshops, can help to ensure that students stay on track and complete their programmes.

Ultimately, fostering a supportive and inclusive learning environment is crucial to improving student retention. By focusing on these key areas and adopting a comprehensive, collaborative approach, higher education institutions can better support their students, reduce attrition, and ensure that higher education remains both accessible and effective for all individuals, regardless of their background or circumstances. This will not only benefit students but also contribute to the development of a more educated, skilled workforce and society as a whole.

References

Astin, A. W. (1984). Student involvement: A developmental theory for higher education. *Journal of College Student Personnel, 25*(4), 297–308.

Astin, A. W. (1999). Student involvement: A developmental theory for higher education. *Journal of College Student Development, 40*(5), 518–529.

Bailey, T. R., Jeong, D. W., & Cho, S. W. (2010). Referral, enrolment, and completion in developmental education sequences in community colleges. *Economics of Education Review, 29*(2), 255–270. https://doi.org/10.1016/j.econedurev.2009.09.002.

Bastable, S. B. (2008). *Nursing education: Foundations for practice excellence* (2nd ed.). Jones and Bartlett Publishers.

Benner, P., Sutphen, M., Leonard, V., & Day, L. (2010). *Educating nurses: A call for radical transformation.* Jossey-Bass.

Cant, R. P., & Cooper, S. J. (2010). Simulation-based learning in nurse education: A systematic review. *Journal of Advanced Nursing, 66*(1), 3–15. https://doi.org/10.1111/j.1365-2648.2009.05114.x.

Crombie, A., Brindley, J., Harris, D., Marks-Maran, D., & Thompson, T. M. (2013). Factors that enhance rates of completion: What makes students stay? *Nurse Education Today, 33*(11), 1282–1287. https://doi.org/10.1016/j.nedt.2013.03.020.

Crombie, D., Housego, S., McCaffrey, G., & Jakes, R. (2013). Stress and coping in nursing students. *Journal of Advanced Nursing, 69*(1), 167–174. https://doi.org/10.1111/j.1365-2648.2012.06090.x.

Deci, E. L., & Ryan, R. M. (1985). *Intrinsic motivation and self-determination in human behavior.* Springer Science & Business Media.

DeWitt, L. A., & Carr, E. C. (2015). The role of faculty in promoting nursing student retention and engagement: Supporting motivation through teaching. *Nursing Education Perspectives, 36*(1), 42–47. https://doi.org/10.5480/13-1265.

Eick, S. A., Williamson, G. R., & Heath, V. (2012). A systematic review of placement-related attrition in nurse education. *International Journal of Nursing Studies, 49*(10), 1299–1309. https://doi.org/10.1016/j.ijnurstu.2011.12.004.

Engle, J., & Tinto, V. (2008). *Moving beyond access: College success for low-income, first-generation students.* Pell Institute for the Study of Opportunity in Higher Education.

Fredricks, J. A., Blumenfeld, P. C., & Paris, A. H. (2004). School engagement: Potential of the concept, state of the evidence. *Review of Educational Research, 74*(1), 59–109. https://doi.org/10.3102/00346543074001059.

Glossop, C. (2002). Student nurse attrition: Use of an exit-interview procedure to determine students' leaving reasons. *Nurse Education Today, 22*(5), 375–386. https://doi.org/10.1054/nedt.2001.0724.

Goldrick-Rab, S. (2016). *Paying the price: College costs, financial aid, and the betrayal of the American dream.* University of Chicago Press.

Hossler, D., Ziskin, M., & Gross, J. P. K. (2009a). Getting serious about institutional performance in student retention: Research-based lessons on effective policies and practices. *About Campus, 13*(6), 2–11. https://doi.org/10.1002/abc.267.

Hossler, D., Ziskin, M., & Gross, J. P. K. (2009b). The role of financial aid in improving college access and success. *The Journal of College Student Retention: Research, Theory & Practice, 10*(3), 227–250. https://doi.org/10.2190/CS.10.3.b.

Jeffreys, M. R. (2007). Tracking students through program entry, progression, graduation, and licensure: Assessing undergraduate nursing student retention and success. *Nurse Education Today, 27*(5), 406–419. https://doi.org/10.1016/j.nedt.2006.07.003.

Jones, J., & Watt, J. (2011). The impact of external motivations on nursing student engagement and retention. *Nurse Education Today, 31*(1), 19–24. https://doi.org/10.1016/j.nedt.2010.04.013.

Kuh, G. D. (2009). *Assessing student engagement in college: A guide for faculty and administrators.* National Institute for Learning Outcomes Assessment.

Kuh, G. D., Kinzie, J., Buckley, J. A., Bridges, B. K., & Hayek, J. C. (2007). *Piecing together the student success puzzle: Research, propositions, and recommendations. ASHE Higher Education Report, 34(6).* Wiley Periodicals.

Kuh, G. D., Kinzie, J., Schuh, J. H., & Whitt, E. J. (2008). *Student success in college: Creating conditions that matter.* John Wiley & Sons.

Lockhart, S., & DeLuca, P. (2019). Factors influencing retention in nursing education: Understanding student persistence. *Nurse Education Today, 79*, 30–38. https://doi.org/10.1016/j.nedt.2019.04.015.

Luthans, F., & Youssef, C. M. (2007). *Positive organizational behavior: An evidence-based approach.* Sage Publications.

McDonald, K., Mann, C., & O'Byrne, P (2016). Peer mentorship in nursing programs: A strategy for success. *Nursing Education Perspectives, 37*(2), 88–91. https://doi.org/10.1097/01.NEP.0000000000000191.

Pascarella, E. T., & Terenzini, P. T. (2005). *How college affects students: A third decade of research (Vol. 2).* Jossey-Bass.

Ryan, R. M., & Deci, E. L. (2000). Self-determination theory and the facilitation of intrinsic motivation, social development, and well-being. *American Psychologist, 55*(1), 68–78. https://doi.org/10.1037/0003-066X.55.1.68.

Schunk, D. H., Pintrich, P. R., & Meece, J. L. (2008). *Motivation and learning: Theory and research.* Pearson Education.

Seidman, A. (2005). *College student retention: Formula for student success.* Rowman & Littlefield.

Shaw, T. (2018). Engagement and retention in nursing programs: The role of community and connection. *Journal of Nursing Education, 57*(1), 46–50. https://doi.org/10.3928/01484834-20180122-02.

Sinclair, M., Hassett, P., & Dunn, S. (2015). The influence of intrinsic motivation on nursing student retention: A focus on the nursing profession. *Journal of Nursing Education, 54*(2), 74–80. https://doi.org/10.3928/01484834-20150122-03.

Swail, W. S., Redd, K. E., & Perna, L. W. (2003). Retaining minority students in higher education: A framework for success. *ASHE-ERIC Higher Education Report, 30*(2), 1–104.

Tinto, V. (1993). *Leaving college: Rethinking the causes and cures of student attrition* (2nd ed.). University of Chicago Press.

Tinto, V. (2012). *Completing college: Rethinking institutional action.* University of Chicago Press.

CHAPTER 3

Key Findings of the Attrition Research Project

Amanda Costello

Background

Evidence suggests that learners may not engage with their programme of study and do not always take advantage of the support available to them. Further nuances from the research demonstrate that learners who are experiencing difficulties and struggling with their programme are most at risk of transient levels of stress and low motivation and engagement. Research data of the lived experiences of undergraduate nursing learner voices are explicit regarding the perceived pressure of work, especially preparing for and completing assessments while developing professional knowledge, skills, and attitudes. Consequently, learners may leave their programme of study for a range of reasons unknown to the academic team at the time of withdrawal or may experience unsuccessful assessment leading to fail and finish decisions at progression and award examination boards.

Consequently, RePAIR funding projects, awarded by a Northwest England funding project, were implemented to support the planning, development, and implementation of high-impact actions and interventions to reduce attrition and improve retention for learners of pre-registration nursing, midwifery, and allied health professions across the Northwest of England.

Successful organisations have been selected for their creative and innovative approaches to improve the support and retention of those in priority programmes and/or professions with the highest levels of attrition, and/or from underrepresented groups across settings, sectors, and professions.

This Northwest England research project presents a detailed, idiographic examination of how participants make sense of their experiences as undergraduate nurses at risk of attrition, via semistructured interviews. The project aimed to explore any challenges that learners navigated regarding their own risk of attrition. It aspired to gain insight into participants' individual stories and how these influence change within their own learning journeys. Listening to participants and the idiosyncratic ways they understand and ascribe meaning to their social and professional worlds as undergraduate nurses was at the heart of the research. The research includes a Maths for Nurses pilot intervention and examines the undergraduate nurses' starting points, as well as formative and summative assessment progress.

A narrative review of the literature was undertaken using the Preferred Reporting Items for Systematic reviews and Meta-Analyses (PRISMA) guideline to understand the attrition issues better. Studies undertaken between 2010 and 2023 were included. Four themes were identified from the narrative reviews and included conceptualising attrition using theories; placement, academic, and course-related issues; personal circumstances, including a subtheme of challenges for male pre-registration students; and support and coping strategy. The narrative reviews explored the multifactorial nature of attrition among undergraduate nursing students.

The second element of the study involved the Maths for Nurses pilot intervention project and included an exploration of the lived experiences of undergraduate nursing students about their studies. Qualitative data were collected and analysed along with an assessment of students' learning and performance based on the baseline, formative, and summative assessments. From the qualitative findings, seven themes emerged including (1) Barriers to learner engagement, (2) Additional support, (3) Intervention and engagement, (4) Successful learning, (5) Sense of self, (6) Learner at risk beliefs, and (7) Relationship beliefs and practice. The findings indicate that students experience myriad challenges while undertaking their undergraduate nursing programmes, and when they are given the right support, they are motivated to stay on and complete their nursing programmes to contribute to the healthcare workforce. In addition, students are pleased with the existing and new intervention groups, such as Leap Online, Maths for Nurses, and Academic Writing Skills groups. These skills are necessary given recent issues with medication safety and errors that could have resulted from poorly trained nurses and healthcare workforces. For instance, the impact on the health of patients and on the staff involved in such errors is significant both financially and emotionally. The evidence suggests that more intervention groups are needed with a consistent approach and planning for a 'business as usual' approach, to ensure that the gains made from the intervention project are maintained for current and future students. Evidence suggests that the intervention strategies will improve their engagement with their studies, improve their mathematics skills, and enable them to go on to complete their programmes successfully.

Introduction

The role of nurses has been consistently highlighted as being critical to the functioning of both hospital and community health services, similar to that of other healthcare professionals (Alvarez et al., 2019). Establishing a robust and nurturing environment within higher education institutions (HEIs) is likewise seen as essential for developing such vital skills compared to other professional fields (Hamshire et al., 2019; Ifenthaler & Yau, 2020). However, the persistent issue of attrition in nursing education presents a stark contrast considering the emphasis on motivation and engagement, yet it has not been adequately addressed, as Urwin et al. (2010) observed. The complex nature of this issue is further complicated by the fact that it is not driven by a single factor, but by a confluence of circumstances similarly affecting student retention.

Moreover, research has consistently identified demographic factors such as gender, ethnicity, and disability as potential catalysts for attrition (Bolton & Lewis, 2025; Hubble et al., 2025). In the same way, the unique pressures faced by nursing students, including financial burdens and the balance between academic and practical demands, further complicate their educational journey (Tufano et al., 2023). Yet, while the UK provides valuable case studies, a broader international perspective is crucial, reflecting the universal scope of healthcare challenges. Therefore the narrative review, utilising the Sample, Phenomenon of Interest, Design, Evaluation, and Research type (SPIDER) tool, aimed to bridge the knowledge gap with an international outlook, considering the variety of factors associated with noncompletion and the diverse support systems available.

As vital players in the healthcare system, nurses face the pressures of clinical duties and the challenge of navigating the rigorous demands of their training. In contrast, the nurturing potential of HEIs is often marred by the phenomenon of student burnout, a growing concern that demands academic scrutiny (see Chapter 1). Similarly, reviews by Burleson et al. (2023) and Arian et al. (2023) have explored nursing student burnout, its prevalence, and interventions, highlighting the multifaceted nature of its causes. Likewise, Liu et al. (2023) illuminate the retention difficulties faced by regional, rural, and remote undergraduate nursing students in Australia, adding to the complexity by focusing on environmental and sociocultural factors.

In an effort to address this gap, the review utilises the SPIDER tool to synthesise findings from various studies, including the prevalence and mitigation of burnout as identified by Burleson et al. (2023) and Arian et al. (2023), alongside the retention challenges documented by Liu et al. (2023). This narrative approach was considered more appropriate to a systematic review, as it aimed to forge a comprehensive understanding of the multifaceted issues influencing nursing education, thus contributing to a more global discourse on the subject. In this way the review not only consolidated existing knowledge but also highlighted areas where further research was needed to develop effective strategies for reducing attrition and supporting nursing students, thereby fostering a more resilient future nursing workforce.

NARRATIVE LITERATURE REVIEW

The literature review utilised the SPIDER tool to formulate the review question and ensure the comprehensive coverage of key concepts related to attrition among pre-registration and nursing students. Keywords were derived from the research question, encompassing the concepts of attrition, pre-registration, nurses, and students. Boolean operators (OR, AND) combined these terms to generate a relevant and productive search strategy using databases such as CINAHL-EBSCO and PubMed/MEDLINE. Additionally, Google Scholar was utilised to search grey literature and unpublished works. A hand search of abstracts from the reviewed articles was also conducted to identify relevant literature. Although a narrative

TABLE 3.1 ■ **Keywords and Concepts**

Key Concepts	Attrition	Pre-registration	Students
Keywords	"attrition" "dropout"	"nurses" "pre-registration"	"students"

TABLE 3.2 ■ **Inclusion and Exclusion Criteria**

Inclusion Criteria	Exclusion Criteria
• **Studies published between 2010 and 2024:** This criterion ensures that the review would include recent research and allowed for an exploration of factors associated with attrition within a relevant timeframe. • **Peer-reviewed and primary research:** Including only peer-reviewed studies ensures the selection of rigorous and credible research, while focusing on primary research ensures that the review is based on original data. • **Qualitative, quantitative, and mixed methods research designs:** Encompassing various research designs allows for a comprehensive understanding of the factors contributing to attrition, considering both qualitative insights and quantitative evidence. • **Papers involving attrition among pre-registration students (nurses, midwives, and physiotherapists):** Limiting the review to papers specifically addressing attrition among pre-registration students in healthcare programmes ensures the relevance and applicability of the findings to the target population. • **Papers written in English:** Including only English-language papers facilitates comprehension and accessibility for the review team and potential readers.	• **Papers not involving pre-registration students:** Excluding studies that do not focus on pre-registration students ensures the alignment of the selected studies with the research question and population of interest. • **Papers not written in English:** Excluding studies written in languages other than English eliminates potential language barriers and ensures efficient comprehension and analysis by the review team. • **Studies published before 2010 or after 2024:** Setting a specific timeframe for inclusion helps to maintain the review's focus on recent research and ensures the examination of factors relevant to the contemporary context. • **Papers that are not peer reviewed or primary research:** Excluding non–peer-reviewed studies and secondary research ensures the selection of high-quality primary research that contributed original insights to the understanding of attrition among healthcare students. • **Papers unrelated to attrition among healthcare students:** Excluding studies that do not directly address attrition among healthcare students avoids potential inclusion of irrelevant research, maintaining the focus and relevance of the review.

literature review was undertaken, the PRISMA guideline was applied to select papers that met the inclusion criteria to add rigour and transparency to the process. See Table 3.1.

INCLUSION AND EXCLUSION CRITERIA

The inclusion criteria of the literature review focused on studies published between 2010 and 2024 to investigate the factors contributing to attrition among healthcare students and to assess the effects of interventions implemented by HEIs and policymakers. This timeframe was chosen to enable a comprehensive exploration of attrition-related factors and the impact of initiatives aimed at creating a supportive learning environment for students See Table 3.2. By considering studies within this

TABLE 3.3 ■ **Workshop Attendance in November and December 2022**

Date	Number of Participants
November–December 2022	
8 November	20
15 November	16
22 November	17
29 November	21
6 December	17

specific period, the review aimed to provide a contemporary understanding of the factors influencing attrition rates and the effectiveness of strategies implemented by HEIs and policymakers. This approach ensured that the review captured recent developments in the field and accounted for the changing landscape of healthcare education. The selected timeframe facilitated an in-depth examination of attrition among healthcare students and the measures undertaken to address this issue.

Following the application of inclusion and exclusion criteria, 13 studies were included in the review. These criteria encompassed papers published between 2010 and 2024: peer-reviewed primary research articles employing qualitative, quantitative, or mixed methods designs, and studies focusing on attrition among pre-registration students, including nurses and physiotherapists. Papers that did not involve pre-registration students or were not written in English were excluded from the review. By incorporating various databases and conducting a hand search, efforts were made to minimise selection bias and capture a wide range of primary research articles. However, it is important to acknowledge the limitations of the review, including the exclusion of non-English papers and the potential omission of relevant contributions from policy documents, guidance, and grey literature. See Table 3.3.

RESULTS AND FINDINGS

The narrative review includes 13 studies across different countries. The countries contributing to the review were the UK (n = 7), Spain (n = 1), South Africa (n = 1), the Netherlands (n = 1), and the United States (n = 3). The research methods utilised in these studies include mixed methods (n = 2), qualitative (n = 1), quantitative (n = 9), and documentary evidence (n = 1). The review identified the following themes: conceptualising attrition using theories; placement, academic, and course-related issues; personal circumstances, with a subtheme of challenges for male pre-registration students; and support and coping strategy. These themes highlight the multifaceted nature of attrition among pre-registration students in healthcare programmes.

Theme 1: Using Theory to Conceptualise Issues With Attrition Among Nursing Students

In examining attrition among nursing students, Hamshire et al. (2019) employed the wicked problem theory to address this phenomenon's intricate and multifaceted

TABLE 3.4 ■ **Number of Participants in the Maths for Nurses Workshop From January to May 2023**

Date	Number of Participants
3 January	10
10 January	14
17 January	16
24 January	12
31 January	14
7 February	17
14 February	18
21 February	20
28 February	20
7 March	21
14 March	21 and 23 (two groups)
21 March	20 and 19 (two groups)
28 March	22 (formative exam)
4 April	18
11 April	20
18 April	21
25 April	20 (summative Medicine Management exam, 80% pass mark)
9 May	1

nature. Their utilisation of this theoretical lens exemplifies a sophisticated and comprehensive approach required to comprehend the root causes of attrition and develop viable and innovative solutions. The authors put forth the notion that effective management strategies entail the design of flexible curricula that accommodate students' commitments and priorities, alongside implementing responsive clinical placements that allow for open communication between students and staff. Furthermore, Hughes (2013) conducted a meticulous review of student records in midwifery programmes, employing a well-defined theoretical framework to delve into the intricacies of recruitment and selection methods, thus illuminating the factors that contribute to student dropout.

To delve into anxiety and academic procrastination among pre-registration students, the cognitive avoidance theory of worry proposed by Borkovec et al. (2004) was employed. The empirical findings from this investigation emphasise that students who exhibit strong motivation and self-efficacy, coupled with successful academic performance, are less inclined to postpone their academic tasks compared with their struggling counterparts. This analysis draws attention to the importance of addressing the underlying factors that impede academic progress and student motivation to mitigate the risks of attrition effectively See Table 3.4.

Mcdermott et al. (2020) crafted a comprehensive conceptual framework that accentuates the pivotal role of resilience in curbing attrition rates among healthcare students. Their framework elucidates the significance of resilience, as it manifests through diminished depressive symptoms and a positive psychological outlook, which in turn engenders reduced academic distress. Moreover, they found that a supportive campus climate prioritising students' mental health and well-being is a moderating factor in alleviating attrition risks.

As a response to the prevailing attrition challenges, HEIs have implemented a range of strategies. Hughes (2013) and Jinks et al. (2014) point to the utilisation of interviews and competency-based assessments as integral components of the student selection and recruitment process, aiming to bolster the quality of candidates admitted to pre-registration programmes and reduce attrition rates. Additionally, Jones and Spiva (2023) propose the ANCC Outcome-Based Continuing Education (OB-CE) framework, which pertains to healthcare professionals' learning and assessment processes, aligning with the outcome-driven nature of the healthcare domain.

Theme 2: Placement, Academic, and Course-Related Issues

The findings from various studies shed light on the academic and course-related issues contributing to attrition among healthcare students. Ten Hoeve et al. (2017) conducted a longitudinal study. They found that nearly a quarter of nursing students considered withdrawing from the programme, primarily due to dissatisfaction with the educational programme, such as a perceived low academic performance and excessive focus on theoretical learning.

McKeever et al. (2018) reported that students needed to prepare for the level of academic work and felt the need to step up their efforts. Meeting deadlines became challenging due to coursework, clinical placements, and personal pressures. This aligns with the findings of Jinks et al. (2014), who noted that most dropouts occurred in the first year, primarily due to examination failures, but as students progressed into the second year, the number considering leaving dropped to 3%. Wray et al. (2017) investigated factors affecting the completion of pre-registration nursing programmes and found that age at entry played a contrasting role compared to non-nursing programmes. Older students had a lower attrition rate compared to younger students. Additionally, factors such as the location of the participants, entry qualifications, and having dependents were found to significantly impact the completion of pre-registration nursing programmes.

Jinks et al. (2014) reviewed training records from 1955 to 1968 and identified academic failure, personal problems, and unsuitability for a nursing career as reasons for attrition. These studies collectively emphasise the role of academic challenges, programme suitability, and personal circumstances in student attrition. Additionally, understanding students' unique needs and challenges at different stages of their studies and considering the influence of age, location, and personal circumstances can contribute to designing interventions and support systems that promote student retention in pre-registration healthcare programmes.

The investigation into the culture of clinical placements illuminates significant concerns that directly impact attrition rates among healthcare students. The research conducted by Hamshire et al. (2019) unveils a prevalent sentiment among students on placement, wherein they perceive inadequate training due to understaffing, rendering them as healthcare assistants or mere auxiliary support. This unfavourable perception and a lack of substantial learning opportunities become a pivotal consideration for students when contemplating withdrawal from their programmes. Additionally, Kneafsey et al. (2012) brought attention to the students' perceived need for preparedness for placement, specifically regarding training in patient handling. Despite the students' expectations of comprehensive instruction, the reality is that only a minority of practice areas provided sufficient training in moving and handling procedures. This observation spotlights the heightened risk of musculoskeletal injuries among nurses, potentially leading to attrition due to health-related factors as students frequently resort to unsafe manual handling techniques, resulting in physical discomfort and illness.

Theme 3: Personal Circumstances

The existing body of literature sheds light on the various academic and course-related factors contributing to attrition among healthcare students. Jinks et al. (2014) revealed that a significant proportion of students who withdrew from pre-registration nursing programmes did so within the initial year, citing domestic reasons and issues with personal health. Onieva-Zafra et al. (2020) conducted a cross-sectional study and discovered that many nursing students experienced moderate to high levels of perceived stress, with those specialising in areas like emergency departments and intensive care units reporting heightened stress levels. Additionally, students with longer durations of training experienced anxiety owing to the requisite competencies expected during clinical practice placements. To cope with the stress arising from clinical training, students employed problem-solving strategies, sought social support, and employed cognitive coping mechanisms (Kneafsey et al., 2012). In addition, personal circumstances, such as having dependents or residing locally with access to social support, contribute to higher progression and completion rates among students (Wray et al., 2017).

In a quantitative study by Roos et al. (2016) in South Africa, financial difficulties, poor health, and well-being challenges emerged as primary contributors to attrition among nursing students. Most respondents discontinued their pre-registration programmes in year 1, reducing the number of enrolled students at the participating university. Surprisingly, many students who departed from the programme believed that no intervention could have persuaded them to remain. This discrepancy in interpretation deviates from Seidman (2005, 2018) and his definition of attrition, which characterises it as the failure of a student to enrol in consecutive terms. Hughes (2013) further revealed that personal reasons like financial constraints, lack of preparedness, and dissatisfaction with the course and institution are influential factors in students' decisions to withdraw. Financial pressures, particularly for students with childcare responsibilities, and perceived inadequacies in childcare support were additional factors that compelled some students to contemplate leaving their programmes (Hamshire et al., 2019; McKeever et al., 2018).

SUBTHEME 1: CHALLENGES FOR MALE PRE-REGISTRATION STUDENTS

The implications for practice arising from the critical examination of attrition among healthcare students, with a specific focus on male pre-registration nursing students, underscore the importance of addressing the challenges related to gender diversity in the healthcare field. Taylor et al. (2022) highlight the isolation experienced by male students due to the scarcity of visible male role models within educational and clinical settings. This limited exposure to various practice areas and learning opportunities can contribute to attrition among male students. To mitigate this, it is recommended to implement strategies such as providing training programmes for medical and clinical staff to raise awareness of unconscious biases and foster a more inclusive environment. Additionally, incorporating gender diversity into learning materials can help to create an educational atmosphere that supports all students. Although gender was not found to be significantly associated with attrition in the study by Hughes (2013), it is essential to note that the majority of participants were female. This highlights the necessity of adopting an inclusive approach that supports all students, regardless of their gender, in making well-informed career choices and addressing any discrepancies between their expectations and the realities of their educational journey.

Theme 4: Support and Coping Strategy

McKeever et al. (2018) emphasise the importance of targeted interventions and consistent support services in mitigating dropout rates among healthcare students, particularly during the critical first year of their studies. Their findings revealed three prominent themes: the aspiration to pursue a nursing career, prior work experience, and the expectations and preparations related to the nursing profession. Some respondents attributed their resilience and commitment to the course to early exposure to healthcare settings. Furthermore, the duration of enrolment has been shown to play a role in students' resilience, with older students exhibiting higher completion rates than their younger counterparts, likely due to their increased maturity and academic readiness (Wray et al., 2017).

Kneafsey et al. (2012) argue for integrating positive coping strategies within the pre-registration curriculum, advocating for providing effective tools to students before engaging in clinical placements. This proactive approach acknowledges the potential challenges that students may encounter and aims to empower them with suitable coping mechanisms.

In a cross-sectional study conducted by Mcdermott et al. (2020) among nursing students in the United States, resilience was associated with reduced depressive episodes and a positive academic attitude. While a supportive academic environment, particularly regarding mental health and well-being, proved beneficial for students, it is noteworthy that students who perceived a lack of support from their academic environment derived more significant academic benefits from their resilience. The preceding suggests that their resilience served as a protective factor against external challenges.

Discussion

The critical examination of attrition among healthcare students is multifaceted and encompasses various areas of intervention. Using theoretical frameworks can provide valuable insights into the complex nature of attrition. The wicked problem theory employed by Hamshire et al. (2019) highlights the multifactorial nature of attrition and emphasises the need for comprehensive interventions considering both intended and unintended outcomes. Similarly, the application of Walker and Avant's concept analysis technique by Custer sheds light on the factors contributing to test anxiety among nursing students, facilitating the development of targeted strategies such as time management and reducing procrastination.

Addressing the academic challenges faced by students is paramount in mitigating attrition. Effective management of academic pressures, including assignment deadlines and practice placement requirements, is essential for students' success (Carlson, 2015; McKeever et al., 2018). Providing appropriate support during in-class sessions and practice placements, as Hamshire et al. (2019) suggested, can help students to navigate these challenges and maintain engagement with their studies.

Personal circumstances, such as childcare responsibilities, present significant obstacles for many students (Hamshire et al., 2019; McKeever et al., 2018; Wray et al., 2017). Institutions and placement areas must find innovative ways to address these concerns and provide tailored support to enable students to balance their caregiving responsibilities with their academic pursuits. Financial difficulties also emerge as a significant hurdle, particularly for international students and those ineligible for financial support (Roos et al., 2016). Institutions and placement areas should consider providing financial assistance or exploring alternative sources of funding to alleviate the financial burdens faced by students, such as travel and living costs. A critical examination of attrition among healthcare students reveals the need for targeted interventions and support systems that consider the diverse demographic composition of nursing students. Gibson (2014) highlights the predominant presence of female and White students in nursing programmes, whereas Taylor et al. (2022) emphasise the challenges male students face in predominantly female work environments. As a result, there is a need to help create an environment for male students. This will promote maturity and resilience among them to navigate the unique challenges they may encounter.

Ensuring satisfactory clinical placements is crucial in bridging the gap between theory and practice. However, students often report feeling ill prepared for their placement, mainly due to insufficient support and mentorship from healthcare organisations (Kneafsey et al., 2012). Inadequate time spent with practice assessors or supervisors further compounds this issue, limiting the quality of student learning experiences (Ten Hoeve et al., 2017). Consequently, efforts should be made to enhance the support and guidance provided during clinical placements to ensure that students feel adequately prepared and supported. Despite possessing a caring nature and positive clinical experience, poor performance in the second year can undermine students' confidence and lead to doubts about their ability to succeed (Ten Hoeve et al., 2017). Therefore, it is essential to address the psychological impact of academic challenges and provide appropriate interventions to support students in overcoming these obstacles.

Conclusion

This narrative literature review has examined the factors contributing to attrition among nursing and registration students. By employing a conceptual framework such as the wicked problem theory, a comprehensive understanding of the multifaceted nature of attrition has been achieved, enabling targeted interventions to address the issue effectively. The review has identified various reasons students may drop out of their programmes, including academic challenges, placement difficulties, and personal circumstances. Managers in HEIs and clinical placement areas must proactively identify problematic areas that hinder students' learning experiences which may lead to attrition. Additionally, teachers and module planners should carefully consider the scheduling of classes to minimise conflicts with assignment deadlines and placement periods, thereby reducing stress levels among students.

Limitations

The limitations of this narrative review should be acknowledged. The review focused on factors contributing to attrition among healthcare students, drawing from mainly primary research papers. However, it is essential to note that only 13 studies met the inclusion criteria, potentially excluding relevant findings from other high-quality studies. Additionally, the review excluded policy documents, guidance, and evidence from grey literature, which could have provided valuable insights. Furthermore, despite efforts to include articles from other pre-registration programmes, the review included articles from nursing and physiotherapy students, limiting the generalisability of the findings. Using the PRISMA flow diagram provided transparency in the paper selection process, reducing selection bias. Nonetheless, the inclusion criteria requiring studies to be written in English may have excluded valuable contributions published in other languages. These limitations should be considered when interpreting the review findings.

Implication for Practice

Considering the proportion of students who discontinue their pre-registration programmes before completion, it is paramount that interventions targeted at mitigating attrition are initiated promptly upon admission. Such action necessitates the implementation of preprogramme orientation initiatives aimed at providing prospective students with realistic perspectives of the academic and clinical contexts, facilitating informed decision making. Notably, HEIs and clinical practice settings typically offer support services for struggling students; however, the timely dissemination of this vital information is crucial. Moreover, personal tutorial sessions should adopt a proactive approach in directing students towards relevant support services.

Additionally, periodic drop-in sessions should be available to address emotional and mental health concerns.

Placement areas should prioritise comprehensive training and induction programmes before students commence their clinical placements, emphasising proper manual handling techniques to promote safety for students and patients. This proactive stance mitigates potential risks and injuries associated with such tasks. In investigating intricate issues like student attrition, incorporating theoretical frameworks augments the value of the study.

Research Design

Having identified the current evidence from the literature along with the implication for practice mentioned previously, this section is focused on the research design and methodological approach needed to investigate the Northwest England research project. The design was developed for the Northwest England funded research pilot project and examines "How far does a pilot intervention programme accelerate success for learners identified at risk of attrition in the Faculty of Health?" It has detailed the aims, research questions, and ethics adopted throughout the research work on the stories of undergraduate nurses, and their struggles within their studies which may cause them to be at risk of attrition. Evidence showed that learners who have experienced difficulties and have struggled with their programme are the most at risk of transient levels of stress and low motivation and engagement (Alvarez et al., 2019; Lo, 2002). The qualitative data were combined with the assessment results collected at baseline, formative, and summative assessment to provide an understanding of the impact, if any, of the pilot intervention on students' academic performance.

The research design considers the pilot group research questions and explores the ethical framework that has guided the research design using reflexivity from the pilot project.

Research Aim and Research Questions

The aim of this research project is to address why undergraduate nursing students may be at risk of attrition by addressing the following research questions:

1. What are the key barriers stopping learners from engaging with the programme?
2. How do we find out what extra support these learners require?
3. How are the impacts of the intervention programmes making a difference to learner engagement and success?
4. Does intervention support the learner's sense of self and become more agentic?

Design for Data Collection

The researchers chose to use (mixed methods due to the baseline data used for students before they commenced the Maths for Nurses intervention) qualitative research methodologies to investigate, interpret, and describe the social reality of the lived experiences of undergraduate nurses at risk of attrition.

Data would be collected using quantitative and qualitative methods. The combination of qualitative and quantitative methods in a single study is commonly practised and accepted in many areas in healthcare research, with each of the methods based on a paradigm (Sale et al., 2002), whereas a qualitative approach adopts a naturalistic approach to enquiry in a real-world environment to explore the meanings attributed by participants to their experiences, where numeric data with indication of frequency of medical events is often missing (Ritchie & Lewis, 2003).

Interpreting the stories of undergraduate nurses' lived experiences of their struggles during their 3-year nursing programme supported the research process by using the Interpretative Phenomenological Analysis (IPA) framework for interpretation and making sense of the learners' stories. This follows the work of Moran (2000); drawing on Heidegger's work, the IPA researcher "examines how a phenomenon appears, and the analyst is implicated in facilitating and making sense of this appearance" (Smith et al., 2009, p. 28). The quantitative data compared baseline data of maths assessment with postintervention data while the qualitative, semistructured approach to interviewing would be taken to gain detailed insights into 20 undergraduate nursing students' lived experience of their 3-year nursing course and struggles with their studies. Qualitative interviewing has several advantages for the IPA researcher and fits into the researchers' methodological framework. Firstly, in-depth interviews allow researchers to capture the complexities of participants' lived experiences and the meanings they attach to the phenomenon of study (Englander, 2012; Kvale, 2007). Secondly, compared to more structured data collection approaches, qualitative interviews are more likely to give participants the space and freedom to express 'their own perspectives in their own words' (Kvale, 2007, p. 11).

Ethics Consideration

As part of fostering nonexploitative research relationships with the researchers' participants, full and informed consent was obtained from all who took part. Every participant was made aware that their participation in this research project was entirely voluntary and that they had the right to withdraw at any stage of the research process. Participant privacy was of the utmost concern. Participants' names, places of work, colleagues, family members, and other identifiable details such as hometowns have been anonymised throughout this research project via the use of pseudonyms.

Developing the Interview Schedule

The development and implementation of the Northwest England pilot group interviews informed the researchers' decision to use IPA as a tool. The semistructured interview is popular with qualitative researchers, and the findings from the pilot group interviews enabled reflection on the depth of the interview, which did have its limitations. On reflection, this gave the researchers the clarity to explore the use of semistructured interviews for listening to undergraduate nurse participants' stories.

The researchers followed the guidelines outlined by Smith et al. (2009) on schedule development. These guidelines highlight the importance of open, expansive questions which 'do not make too many assumptions about the participant's experiences or concerns, or lead them towards particular answers' (Smith et al., 2009, p. 56).

SAMPLING FOR QUALITATIVE DATA

Having discussed the stages involved in developing a semistructured interview schedule, the researchers moved on to examine the issue of sampling for IPA research methodology. IPA is concerned with quality and depth as opposed to quantity and breadth (Smith & Osborn, 2008). Challenging 'the traditional linear relationship between "number of participants" and value of research', IPA studies focus on a small sample of individuals (Reid et al., 2005, p. 22). It was decided during the design phase of the research project that the rich, nuanced insights gained from semistructured interviews with undergraduate nurse participants would generate enough data to facilitate a detailed and interpretative case-by-case analysis. The researchers chose a sample size of 20 undergraduate nurses to allow for both an in-depth examination of individual undergraduate nurses' accounts and a detailed consideration of the convergences and divergences among the nursing participants. It also meant that if individual undergraduate nurses dropped out of the study, the researchers would still have enough participants to facilitate a detailed analysis. In addition to small sample sizes, IPA researchers endeavoured to recruit 'a fairly homogeneous sample' who will find the topic under investigation meaningful (Smith et al., 2009, p. 49). The research questions are concerned with undergraduate nurses' risk of attrition. The researchers were interested in the ways in which undergraduate nurses make sense of their struggles within their individual learning journey. The participant inclusion criteria the researchers used therefore meant that participants needed to be nurses who were at risk of leaving the programme due to many variables. Consistent with IPA's commitment to the idiographic, it was anticipated that this inclusion criteria would generate a homogeneous sample that could give a contextualised perspective on undergraduate nurses' struggles within their learning.

The researchers chose to focus on the lived experiences of undergraduate nurses and to understand why they may be at risk of attrition.

To recruit a small, homogeneous sample, a self-selecting sampling strategy was used via an advertised pilot intervention group: Maths for Nurses. 'These people are then used as informants to identify, or put researchers in touch with, others who qualify for inclusion, and these, in turn, identify yet others' (Cohen et al., 2011, p. 158). This process is repetitive and accumulative, like snowball sampling once the self-directing has occurred. Snowball sampling is claimed to be a good technique for gaining access to populations that are 'not easily accessible to researchers through other sampling strategies' (Shinebourne, 2011, p. 54). It became clear that the researchers required a sampling strategy that drew on the referrals of participants via an advertisement for Maths for Nurses with a QR code linked to the university-wide system. The self-selected and snowball sampling offered a way forward.

The researchers anticipated that the findings would have some degree of 'theoretical transferability' (Smith et al., 2009, p. 38). It is, however, essential that, as reflexive researchers, they maintained an awareness of the limitations of the sampling strategy. Browne (2005, p. 57) reminds us that no sampling technique is flawless; 'rather advantages and disadvantages are subjective and often based on research precepts of what is right and wrong.' Having explored the sampling strategy used in this investigation, the researchers introduced the participants' demographic characteristics.

THE INTERVIEW PROCEDURE

Before examining the reflexive stance taken during this research project, it is necessary to present a transparent account of the steps taken to collect and analyse the data. What follows is a step-by-step explanation of the research process.

Following ethical approval, the researchers sent self-selecting participants an invitation to be involved in the project. Once a participant confirmed that they would like to be involved in the project, a suitable time and place were arranged for the interview. It was at this stage that participants could opt for either a face-to-face interview or a telephone interview, depending on their preference and availability.

Before starting the interview, participants received a participant information sheet and were allowed to ask any questions. Participants were made aware that their participation in the research project was entirely voluntary and had the right to withdraw at any stage of the research process. Informed consent was obtained, and participants were asked to sign and date a participant consent form. Once this was complete, participants were asked semistructured interview questions. The schedule was used flexibly according to the individual participant's concerns and interests. Each interview lasted for approximately 20 minutes and was recorded using a digital voice recorder via Otter Notes. After the interview, the researcher thanked participants for their involvement and asked them whether there was anything they would like to add. All of the data collected during the interviews was used and stored in accordance with the Data Protection Act 2018. The researcher later transcribed each audio recording using Otter Notes, and the transcripts gave summary keywords and timings of the conversation, which the researchers found helpful.

THE ANALYTIC PROCESS

IPA is an iterative and creative process that involves exploring, commenting on, and interpreting an individual case in detail. By clustering initial a priori themes together using template analysis, superordinate (main) and subordinate (secondary) themes are developed from each transcript and the data set as a whole. During the data analysis phase of this research project, the researchers followed the guidelines set out by IPA researchers Smith et al. (2009). The stages involved in this process (including signposts to illustrative examples from the researchers' analysis) are presented in the following sections.

Smith et al. (2009, p. 81) advise 'the novice embarking on an IPA study for the first time to begin by working closely with the suggested set of steps.' The researchers adhered to the procedure described later and found the suggested phases to be a useful scaffold. Gee (2011, p. 21) observes that as researchers become more confident analysing data in this way, the steps become a 'road map' one studies 'in advance to chart an overview of a planned journey and, along the way, one refers to it to check whether a part of the route already taken is leading in the right direction.'

The research information that follows moves on to consider the findings and most important issues that arose from the researchers' in-depth, semistructured interviews with 20 undergraduate nurses identified as at risk of attrition. It discusses and interprets the superordinate and subordinate themes from the initial a priori themes that emerged from IPA.

SAMPLE RESULTS AND FINDINGS

The research findings were based on seven superordinate themes that emerged from the IPA process: (1) Barriers to learner engagement, (2) Additional support (3) Intervention and engagement, (4) Successful learning, (5) Sense of self, (6) Learner at risk beliefs, and (7) Relationship beliefs and practice. These themes, along with their accompanying subordinate themes, are explored with the aim of providing the reader with a rich account by researchers of the participants' lived experiences. The researchers then discuss the findings of this NHS England research project in light of extant literature and theory concerned with agency, structure, and reflexivity (Costello, 2020).

THEMES AND ANALYTIC COMMENTARY

The findings of the Northwest England research project show how the researchers' accounting of participants' experience of undergraduate nursing has been shaped by structure and agency. However, examination of the data revealed a large degree of heterogeneity among the participants; each participant described mediating and making sense of structural forces and their agentic capacity to act in a different way. IPA of undergraduate nurses' accounts produced seven superordinate themes. These themes were labelled as follows: (1) Barriers to learner engagement, (2) Additional support, (3) Intervention and engagement, (4) Successful learning, (5) Sense of self, (6) Learner at risk beliefs, and (7) Relationships beliefs and practice.

Each of the themes details different aspects of undergraduate nurses' lived experiences and perceptions, using illustrative quotations to highlight the convergences and divergences among participants.

Maths for Nurses Pilot Intervention

The pilot group of nurses involved in the NHS England research project were invited to join a 5-week Maths for Nurses intervention group; the group was advertised for any student nurse learning at the university. The pilot group was self-selecting whether they wanted to take part in the Maths for Nurses intervention group. Twenty out of the 25 nurses interviewed participated in the intervention group. On entry to the Maths for Nurses intervention group, each nurse had a maths baseline assessment. The baseline score served as a starting point for each undergraduate nurse.

Fig. 3.1 shows that 75% of learners performed below average compared to their entry points, with the minimum of GCSE Maths Grade C or above or Progress 8 Level 4 and above or Entry Level 2 Maths and ELTs score. The 5-week period finished on Tuesday 8 December 2022.

Learners completed a survey at the end of the 5-week period. Learners were asked to rate the quality of assessment and teaching and areas of strength and weakness to formulate future learning. The survey aimed to increase confidence in maths and drug calculations for nurses. Learners were asked, at the end of the survey if they needed further support with understanding the medication doses and calculations of tablets and capsules, liquids and injectables, displacement values, dosages, and body weight.

The majority of learners who participated in the survey said that their maths confidence had increased during the 5-week period. Some learners wanted to carry on with the workshop sessions, whilst others were satisfied that they had learnt enough to become proficient in medicine management and were ready for their placements.

From January 2023, each participant was given an additional maths assessment. The assessment process gave teachers the opportunity to understand where differentiation and scaffolding were necessary for learner progression and growth. In May 2023, learners sat their Medicine Management exam. An average of 45 second-year nurses attended the Maths for Nurses intervention workshops from November

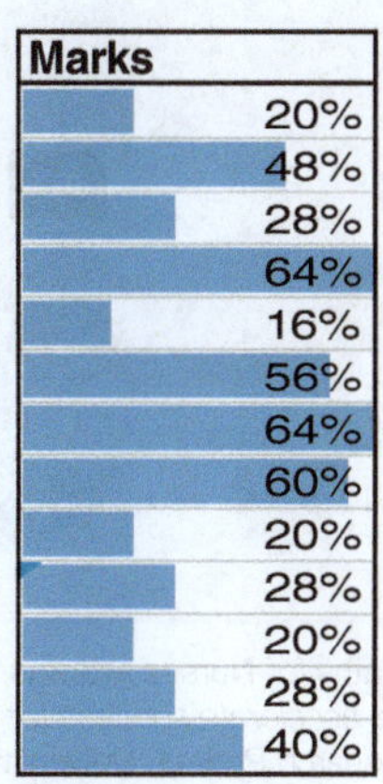

Fig. 3.1 Baseline pilot results. (From Costello, A. J. [2023]. *How far does a pilot intervention programme accelerate success for learners identified at risk of attrition in the faculty of health?* NHS England Funded Research Project, University of Bolton.)

2022 until May 2023; 39 of those learners achieved the 80% pass grade expected in year 2 of the BSc (Hons) Nursing courses, in both direct entry and apprenticeship courses in adult nursing, child nursing, and mental health nursing.

The Maths for Nurses classes continued from June to August 2023; this further included a Maths for Nurses summer school held in August. The feedback from learners has been positive and has led to a strategic plan being implemented to create a standard Maths for Nurses in person and Maths for Nurses online. The offer has been extended to all undergraduate nurses, including the midwifery learners. Furthermore, semester-based maths workshops have been planned and designed to ensure learner confidence and patient safety during placements.

The graph in Fig. 3.2 shows the average initial baseline assessment pass mark of 42% for Maths for Nurses learners in the self-selected pilot.

The formative assessment of 91% is the same Maths for Nurses learners who have sat the Medicine Management exam with the remainder of their peers from the module cohort in year 2 of their undergraduate nursing course. The 86% exam mark is again the same as Maths for Nurses learners who have sat their summative assessment for their Medicine Management final exam. Each learner has the expected learner outcome of the 80% pass mark. Some of the undergraduate nurses who participated in the Maths for Nurses pilot were on their second attempt of their Medicine Management exam and were successful on the second attempt.

The success for the learner has been achieved with a combination of Maths for Nurses intervention learning, Medicine Management module learning, and revision classes within the module (Costello, 2023).

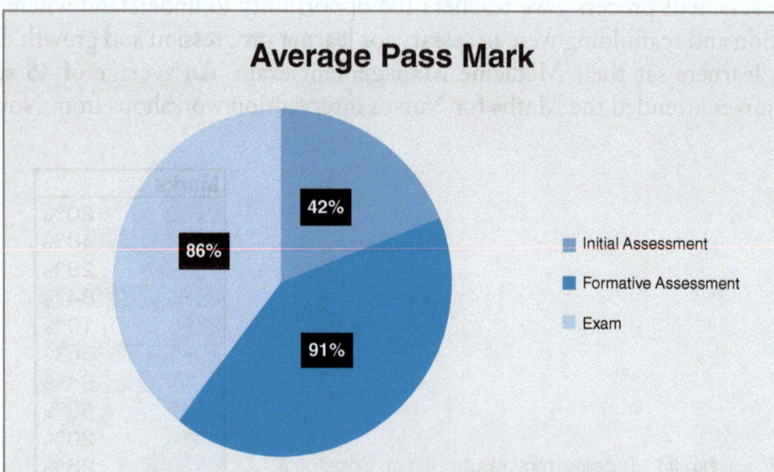

Fig. 3.2 Maths for Nurses average pass mark. (From Costello, A. J. [2023]. *How far does a pilot intervention programme accelerate success for learners identified at risk of attrition in the faculty of health*? NHS England Funded Research Project, University of Bolton.)

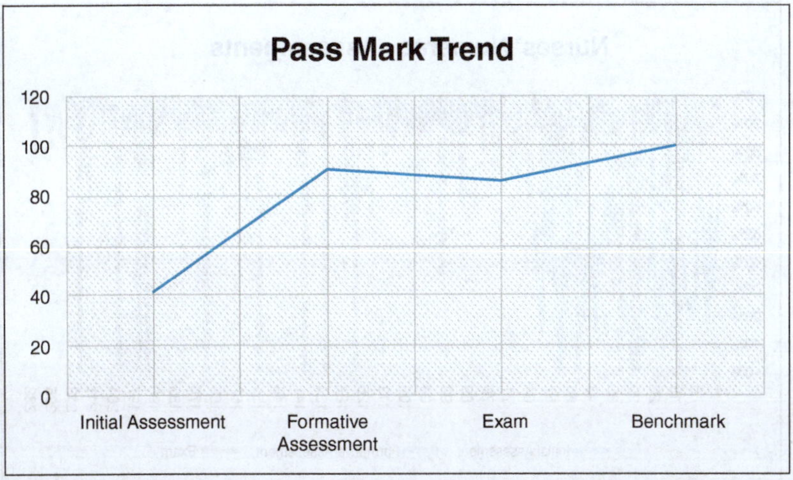

Fig. 3.3 Pass mark trend. (From Costello, A. J. [2023]. *How far does a pilot intervention programme accelerate success for learners identified at risk of attrition in the faculty of health*? NHS England Funded Research Project, University of Bolton.)

The Maths for Nurses pass mark trend in Fig. 3.3 shows the initial baseline at a lower point on the graph, with a steep upward trend, during the Maths for Nurses intervention sessions. The plateauing is due to the undergraduate learner sustaining their new knowledge, understanding, and proficiency at their number and calculation work. The trend chart acts as confidence bands in learner proficiency, and it is observable where the trend line starts to rise again as the learner gains their calculation skills (Costello, 2023).

The graph in Fig. 3.4 demonstrates the level of activity and change developed during the intervention classes. It is also a combination of increased activity during the revision periods for the formative and summative examination with the Medicine Management module. An added dimension to the learning outcome is the peer-to-peer support and one-to-one intervention that supported the differentiation of each undergraduate learner who self-selected on the Maths for Nurses pilot intervention programme (Costello, 2023).

LESSON LEARNT FROM THE MATHS FOR NURSES PILOT INTERVENTION

Medicine Management teaching and learning for undergraduate nursing is designed to teach, practise, and build knowledge and understanding of medicine management skills and ensure patient safety (Weeks et al., 2000). It has been identified that some learners require additional support to enable the learner to pass their Medicine Management exam in years 1, 2, and 3. According to Stelzer et al. (2019), the teaching of medicine management within practice is not enough, and therefore teaching of ordinary computational skills, such as addition, subtraction, multiplication, and division of whole numbers, decimals and fractions,

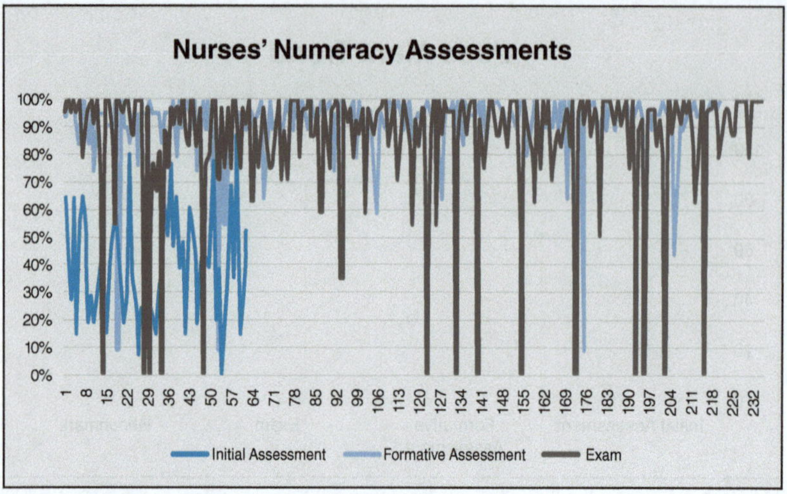

Fig. 3.4 Initial assessment and formative and summative assessments. (From Costello, A. J. [2023]. *How far does a pilot intervention programme accelerate success for learners identified at risk of attrition in the faculty of health*? NHS England Funded Research Project, University of Bolton.)

and conversions between decimals and fractions, are essential skills for learner competence and patient safety. Procedural knowledge needs to be automatic for future practice (Anderson & Schunn, 2000; Ashcraft & Krause, 2007; Daubert & Ramani, 2019).

Maths for Nurses intervention workshops have been successful because they provide learners with the necessary skills and knowledge to perform mathematical calculations accurately and confidently, which is critical for their practice and patient safety. There are several reasons the Maths for Nurses workshop intervention is successful:

- *Builds Confidence*: The Maths for Nurses intervention helps nurses to build confidence in their maths skills, which allows them to perform calculations accurately and efficiently. This confidence also translates into their practice, where they can communicate effectively with colleagues and patients about medication doses and other mathematical calculations.
- *Enhances Safety*: Maths errors can have serious consequences for patient safety. By providing Maths for Nurses intervention workshops, nurses can learn how to perform accurate calculations, which reduces the risk of medication errors and other safety issues.
- *Supports Evidence-Based Practice*: Nurses need to understand and interpret research studies that use mathematical concepts. Maths intervention can provide nurses with the necessary skills to interpret and critically evaluate research studies and make evidence-based decisions in their practice.
- *Personalised Learning*: Maths intervention can be tailored to individual learning styles and needs, which allows nurses to learn at their own pace and in a way that suits them best.

Overall, Maths for Nurses intervention workshops have been successful because they have helped nurses to develop the necessary mathematical skills to provide safe, effective, evidence-based care to their patients. This is more important due to the issues of medication errors and safety issues which are responsible for adverse health incidents and litigation costs for the NHS.

Discussion

In our university, two of the main reasons that students failed to progress with the undergraduate nursing programme are failure at examination and practice placement. This resulted in two flagship intervention programmes to assist students in mitigating the reasons adduced previously. The research project has identified undergraduate nursing learners at risk of not completing their chosen course within the Health and Wellbeing Faculty at the university. Our evidence suggests that learners may not engage with their programme of study and do not take advantage of the support available to them. However, there is encouraging development based on findings from the current study and students' engagement with the Maths for Nurses pilot intervention project.

During the first year, it is important that students have the required numeracy and communication skills to promote safe patient care. For instance, proficiency in their mathematics skills would enable them to accurately calculate the correct doses of medication and avoid medication error; this improves outcomes both at assessment and at clinical placements. This is important given the many medication errors seen among nurses with consequences on the quality of patients' care and avoidable mortalities in some cases (Elliott et al., 2021).

The 'lightbulb moments' experienced by participants can be aligned with the research findings of McKeever et al. (2018), whereby they emphasise targeted intervention to be critical in the first year of learning. In their findings, they revealed prominent themes amongst undergraduate nurses such as an 'aspiration to pursue a nursing career', prior work experience, and the 'expectations and preparations' related to the nursing profession.

Kneafsey et al. (2012) discuss the importance of 'bridging the gap' between theory and placement and preparing students for their clinical practice, which again can give students a good taste of what to expect during their programme. A positive first-year experience could be the motivation that students need to get them through the rest of the programme, as Borkovec et al. (2004) noted as part of their research findings, that students who exhibit strong motivation and self-efficacy, coupled with successful academic performance, are able to complete their studies compared to those who may struggle.

According to Hamshire et al. (2019) and Ifenthaler and Yau (2020), successful completion of university programmes depends on motivation, class attendance, active learning, and being socially embedded within the setting. Accordingly, Carlson (2015) and McKeever et al. (2018) noted that effective management of academic pressures, including assignment deadlines and placement requirements, are essential for learner success. Providing appropriate support during in-class sessions and practice placements, as suggested by Hamshire et al. (2019), can help learners to navigate these challenges and maintain engagement with their undergraduate nursing studies.

Jinks et al. (2014) revealed that a significant proportion of students who withdrew from pre-registration nursing programmes did so within the initial year, citing domestic reasons and issues with personal health. In a further quantitative study by Roos et al. (2016) in South Africa, financial difficulties, poor health, and well-being challenges emerged as primary contributors to attrition among nursing students.

Our findings also suggest that students contend with myriad personal issues such as finance, childcare, and ill health during their studies and would require good support to enable them to complete their programme. This was summed up by Hughes (2013), who explains that 'personal reasons', 'financial constraints', lack of 'preparedness', and 'dissatisfaction' with the course can be factors in students' decisions to withdraw from a course, such as undergraduate nursing, where the variables that Hughes (2013) discusses come into play.

Research undertaken by Hamshire et al. (2019) states that undergraduate nurses who perceive their placements to be inadequate due to understaffing and lack of support can 'contemplate' withdrawing from their programmes. Taylor et al. (2022) further explains the challenges faced by male nurses in predominately female work environments, making it clear that male nurses need to demonstrate a level of maturity and resilience to be able to 'navigate' the challenges that they may experience.

Carlson (2015) and McKeever et al. (2018) state clearly that addressing the academic challenges faced by learners is paramount in mitigating attrition. Research findings by Glogowska et al. (2007) give evidence of how learners' academic work can be affected by negative experiences due to a variety of challenges that affect the completion of assessment work and clinical practice, and is further impacted by financial difficulties and childcare issues. These research findings resonate with the participant voice in Costello (2023, p. 45): 'Learners at risk of attrition whilst undertaking an undergraduate nursing programme.'

The findings indicate that students experience their clinical practice placement differently and devise coping mechanisms aimed at building motivation and resilience to remain and do well in both theory and practice. Early experience of failure and academic challenge can affect learners' university experience. Challenges of academic work were also reported in research findings by Glogowska et al. (2007), who stated that other factors affecting students' completion include negative experiences during clinical placement; challenges of academic work; difficulties with finances, childcare, and lack of and/or inadequate support; and negative experience early in the programme.

Although UK-based students are eligible for financial support during their studies, many respondents felt that the money is not enough to meet their living expenses, with many students engaged in extra work to assist with their financial costs. This view is in line with survey of students by the Office for National

Statistics (2023), where more than half (58%) of those surveyed indicated that their loans were not enough to meet the cost of their living, and a quarter (25%) said that their loans only just covered their living costs. Roos et al. (2016) see financial constraints as a 'major hurdle' affecting especially international students and learners eligible for financial support. The struggles that students experience with the cost of living is even more pronounced among international students, who rarely if ever receive institutional financial support due to their legal status. Students indicate that their inability to meet their financial obligations is putting a lot of strain on their mental health (Frampton, 2022). There is a need for better awareness of where students can assess support services including financial and other areas of needs, as findings from a survey of students indicate varied awareness of financial supports and other forms of assistance, with such variations marked among students from ethnic minority backgrounds in the UK (Office for National Statistics, 2023). For that reason, Roos et al. (2016) suggest that universities need to support their students with financial guidance and signposting to the appropriate services.

Findings from the qualitative data indicate that students who speak English as their second language face challenges navigating their lectures and the assessments to ensure they meet their learning outcomes due to language barriers. This part of the findings aligns with the work of Ashifa (2022), who asserts that students' ability to thrive and survive is impeded by the language barriers that affect communication during their studies.

Glogowska et al. (2007) noted from their studies that 'commitment' to their chosen profession, 'determination', and 'formal and informal support' can determine if students stay to complete their programmes. According to Glogowska et al. (2007, p. 28), 'while most preregistration students went on to complete their programme, some students failed to stay on their course to graduation.' Further discussion with Participant N gave insights into how other nursing students were lacking in motivation due to failed assessments and placements on their first and second attempts. Bakker et al. (2020), Rathnayake and Ekanayaka (2016), and Rudman and Gustavsson (2011) all emphasise in their studies that unsuccessful assessment practice and placement issues have evidence of age and gender as some of the recurrent themes associated with noncompletion of a registration programme. Further evidence cited by the authors suggests challenges experienced by learners such as those around mental health, depressive symptoms, anxiety, burnout, and stress. This information illustrates Participant N's perception that being a nursing student is difficult to maintain if someone is struggling with assessment knowledge and understanding that at times has led to assessment failure.

Borkovec et al. (2004) explain their empirical findings on student learning, stating that students who exhibit strong motivation and self-efficacy, coupled with successful academic performance, are less inclined to postpone their academic tasks compared to their struggling counterparts. This demonstrates the importance of assisting students to address underlying factors that hinder academic progress and student motivation to mitigate the risks of attrition effectively.

The researchers have found the participants' interviews difficult, highlighting the need for further intervention in terms of access to teaching and learning for undergraduate nurses.

Limitations

The study consists of qualitative data and performance data of nursing students which gave a more holistic explanation of the Maths for Nurses pilot intervention. A limitation of this study is that the researchers' sample consists entirely of Black, Asian, and Minority Ethnic (BAME) and White women, both mature and young, and those with a disability learning contract, and only a small sample of BAME and White men. While the idiographic nature of this research project means that any conclusions at which the researchers arrive will be tentative and unable to be generalised, the researchers are quite conscious that the views of BAME and White mature, young, and disabled women cannot be taken to be representative of all women (Crenshaw, 2010). Interpretive phenomenology (IPA) is a methodology that focuses on the particular stories of undergraduate nurses.

Conclusion

Further evidence shows that learners who are experiencing difficulties and struggling with their programme are the most at risk of transient levels of stress and low motivation and engagement. This is due to the perceived pressure of work, especially preparing for and completing assessments while developing professional knowledge, skills, and attitudes.

For students, a variety of reasons can contribute to stress and anxiety. For instance, findings suggest that students perceived being a nursing student as difficult to maintain if struggling with assessment knowledge and understanding, which at times has led to assessment failure.

In addition, some participants explain that childcare, domestic violence, attending the family court, and financial difficulties can make learning impossible. The risk of attrition is high for these learners, and their individual struggles have meant not passing exams and having referrals in all types of assessment. Other divergences and convergences are space, time, lack of understanding, and the need for face-to-face learning.

'Perceived beliefs about staff' have produced findings relating to planning, preparation, and assessment rubrics. Some participants would prefer small-step learning and more practical-based assessment to support learning and language barriers. It is clear from the participants' interview transcripts that they have appreciated the existing intervention groups, such as Leap Online, Maths for Nurses, and Academic Writing Skills groups. The evidence suggests that more intervention groups are needed with a consistent approach and planning for a 'business as usual' approach. A lack of support can lead to undergraduate nursing learner attrition.

Recommendations

- Continue the Maths for Nurses intervention groups both in person and online with a maths lecturer employed on a variable contract by the university. The 'business as usual' approach will be evaluated each semester.
- Continue to collaborate with Leap Live university services to support literacy across the undergraduate nursing programmes, including a spring and summer school to further accelerate learning and to include new nursing cohorts.
- Consider creche facilities as a pilot intervention by applying for external funding against the findings of the attrition project.
- Provide direct support in accessing financial assistance via an information booklet produced by the university.

References

Alvarez, H. A. O., Provencio-Vasquez, E., Slavich, G. M., Laurent, J. G. C., Browning, M., McKee-Lopez, G., Robbins, L., & Spengler, J. D. (2019). Stress and Health in Nursing Students: The Nurse Engagement and Wellness Study. *Nursing Research, 68*(6), 453–463. [Online]. https://doi.org/10.1097/NNR.0000000000000383.

Anderson, J. R., & Schunn, C. D. (2000). Implications of the ACT-R learning theory: No magic bullets. In R. Glasier (Ed.), *(2000) Advances in Instructional Psychology. Vol 5: Educational Design and Cognitive Science* (pp. 1–33). Mahwah, NJ: Lawrence Erlbaum Associates.

Arian, M., Jamshidbeigi, A., Kamali, A., Dalir, Z., & Ali-Abadi, T. (2023). The prevalence of burnout syndrome in nursing students: A systematic review and meta-analysis. *Teaching and Learning in Nursing, 18*(4), 512–520. [Online]. https://doi.org/10.1016/j.teln.2023.04.015.

Ashcraft, M. H., & Krause, J. A. (2007). Working memory, math performance, and math anxiety. *Psychonomic Bulletin & Review, 14*, 243–248. [Online]. https://doi.org/10.3758/BF03194059. [Accessed 6 November 2023].

Ashifa, K. M. (2022). Language Challenges Faced By International Students In Turkey. *Webology, 19*(2), 1762–1767.

Bakker, E. J. M., Kox, J. H. A. M., Boot, C. R. L., Francke, A. L., Beek, A. J.van der, & Roelofs, P. D. D. M. (2020). Improving mental health of student and novice nurses to prevent dropout: A systematic review. *Journal of Advanced Nursing, 76*(10), 2494–2509.

Bolton, P., & Lewis, J. (2025). Equality of access and outcomes in higher education In England. *House of Commons Library Research Briefings, 9195*. [Online]Available from:. https://researchbriefings.files.parliament.uk/documents/CBP-9195/CBP-9195.pdf.

Borkovec, T. D., Alcaine, O. M., & Behar, E. (2004). Avoidance Theory of Worry and Generalized Anxiety Disorder. In R. G. Heimberg, C. L. Turk, & D. S. Mennin (Eds.), *(2004) Generalized Anxiety Disorder: Advances in Research and Practice* (pp. 77–108). New York: Guildford Press.

Browne, K. (2005). Snowball sampling: using social networks to research non-heterosexual women. *International Journal of Social Research Methodology, 8*(1), 47–60.

Burleson, S., Thomas, L., & DeBoor, S. (2023). Effective Interventions for Nursing Student Burnout: A Scoping Review. *Nurse educator, 48*(3), E85–E89. [Online]. https://doi.org/10.1097/NNE.0000000000001348.

Carlson, J. S. (2015). Factors Influencing Retention Among Part-Time Clinical Nursing Faculty. *Nursing Education Perspectives, 36*(1), 42–45. [Online]. https://doi.org/10.5480/13-1231.

Cohen, L., Manion, L., & Morrison, K. (2011). *Research Methods in Education* (7th edn). London: Routledge.

Costello, A. J. (2020). *Stories of female special school headteachers and their experience of headship: an interpretive phenomenological analysis.* Doctoral, Sheffield Hallam University.

Costello, A. J. (2023). *How far does a pilot intervention programme accelerate success for learners identified at risk of attrition in the faculty of health?* NHS England Funded Research Project, University of Bolton.

Crenshaw, K. W. (2010). Close Encounters of Three Kinds: On Teaching Dominance Feminism and Intersectionality. *Tulsa Law Review, 46*(1), 151–189.

Daubert, E. N., & Ramani, G. B. (2019). Math and Memory in Bilingual Preschoolers: the Relations Between Bilingualism, Working Memory, and Numerical Knowledge. *Journal of Cognition and Development, 20*, 314–333. [Online]. https://doi.org/10.1080/15248372.2019.1565536. [Accessed 6 November 2023].

Elliott, R. A., Camacho, E., Jankovic, D., Sculpher, M. J., & Faria, R. (2021). Economic analysis of the prevalence and clinical and economic burden of medication error in England. *BMJ Quality and Safety, 30*(2), 96–105.

Englander, M. (2012). The interview: Data collection in descriptive phenomenological human scientific research. *Journal of Phenomenological Psychology, 43*(1), 13–35.

Frampton, N. (2022). *How the cost of living crisis is affecting students' money and mental health. Money and Mental Health Policy Institute.* [Online] 22 November. Available from:. https://www.moneyandmentalhealth.org/cost-of-living-students/.

Gee, P. (2011). Approach and Sensibility: A Personal Reflection on Analysis and Writing using Interpretive Phenomenological Analysis. *Qualitative Methods in Psychology Bulletin, 11*, 8–22.

Gibson, H. A. (2014). A conceptual view of test anxiety. *Nursing Forum, 49*(4), 267–277. [Online]. https://doi.org/10.1111/nuf.12069.

Glogowaska, M., Young, P., & Lockyer, L. (2007). Should I go or should I stay? A study of factors influencing students' decisions on early leaving. *Active Learning in Higher Education, 8*(1), 63–77.

Hamshire, C., Jack, K., Forsyth, R., Langan, A. M., & Harris, W. E. (2019). The wicked problem of healthcare student attrition. *Nursing Inquiry, 26*(3), 1–8. https://doi.org/10.1111/nin.12294.

Health Equity in England (2020) *The Marmot Review 10 Years On* [Online], Available from: https://www.instituteofhealthequity.org/resources-reports/marmot-review-10-years-on/the-marmot-review-10-years-on-full-report.pdf. [Accessed 27/10/2022].

Hoeve, Y.ten, Castelein, S., Jansen, W. S., Jansen, G. J., & Roodbol, P. F. (2017). Nursing students' changing orientation and attitudes towards nursing during education: A two year longitudinal study. *Nurse Education Today, 48*, 19–24. https://doi.org/10.1016/j.nedt.2016.09.009.

Hubble, S., Bolton, P. and Lewis, J. (2025) *Equality of access and outcomes in higher education in England,* House of Commons Library Research Briefings, 9195.

Hughes, H. A. (2013). Factors influencing attrition rates in midwifery students. *Nursing Standard, 27*(26), 42–48.

Ifenthaler, D., & Yau, J. Y.-K. (2020). Utilising learning analytics to support study success in higher education: a systematic review. *Educational Technology Research and Development, 68*, 1961–1990. https://doi.org/10.1007/s11423-020-09788-z.

Jinks, A. M., Richardson, K., Jones, C., & Kirton, J. A. (2014). Issues concerning recruitment, retention and attrition of student nurses in the 1950/60s: A comparative study. *Nurse Education in Practice, 14*(6), 641–647. https://doi.org/10.1016/j.nepr.2014.07.002.

Jones, N., & Spiva, L. (2023). Nurses Leading Partnership-Driven Transformation to Address the Nursing Shortage. *Journal of Continuing Education in Nursing, 54*(2), 53–55. https://doi.org/10.3928/00220124-20230113-02.

Kneafsey, R., Ramsay, J., Edwards, H., & Callaghan, H. (2012). An exploration of undergraduate nursing and physiotherapy students' views regarding education for patient handling. *Journal of Clinical Nursing, 21*(23-24), 3493–3503. https://doi.org/10.1111/j.1365-2702.2012.04172.x.

Kvale, S. (2007). *Doing Interviews*. London: Sage Publications.

Liu, Z., Xie, Y., Sun, Z., Liu, D., Yin, H., & Shi, L. (2023). Factors associated with academic burnout and its prevalence among university students: a cross-sectional study. *BMC Medical Education, 23*, 317.

Lo, R. (2002). A longitudinal study of perceived level of stress, coping and self-esteem of undergraduate nursing students: an Australian case study. *Journal of Advanced Nursing, 39*(2), 119–126.

Mcdermott, R. C., Fruh, S. M., Williams, S., Hauff, C., Graves, R. J., Melnyk, B. M., & Hall, H. R. (2020). Nursing students' resilience, depression, wellbeing, and academic distress: Testing a moderated mediation model. *Journal of Advanced Nursing, 76*(12), 3385–3397. https://doi.org/10.1111/jan.14531.

McKeever, S., Whiting, L., Anderson, D., & Twycross, A. (2018). Causes of ATtrition in CHIldren's NursinG (CATCHING): An exploratory mixed method study. *Nurse Education in Practice, 32*, 44–51. https://doi.org/10.1016/j.nepr.2018.06.012.

Moran, D. (2000). *Introduction to phenomenology*. Routledge.

Office for National Statistics (2023) *Cost of living and higher education students, England: 30 January to 13 February 2023* [Online], released 24 February 2023.

Onieva-Zafra, M. D., Fernández-Muñoz, J. J., Fernández-Martínez, E., García-Sánchez, F. J., Abreu-Sánchez, A., & Parra-Fernández, M. L. (2020). Anxiety, perceived stress and coping strategies in nursing students: a cross-sectional, correlational, descriptive study. *BMC Medical Education, 20*(1), 1–9. https://doi.org/10.1186/s12909-020-02294-z.

Rathnayake, S., & Ekanayaka, J. (2016). Depression, Anxiety and Stress among Undergraduate Nursing Students in a Public University in Sri Lanka. *International Journal of Caring Sciences, 9*(3), 1020.

Reid, K., Flowers, P., & Larkin, M. (2005). Exploring Lived Experience. *The Psychologist, 18*(1), 20–23.

Ritchie, J., & Lewis, J. (2003). *Qualitative Research Practice: A Guide for Social Science Students and Researchers*. London: Sage Publications.

Roos, E., Fichardt, A. E., MacKenzie, M. J., & Raubenheimer, J. (2016). Attrition of undergraduate nursing students at selected South African universities. *Curationis, 39*(1). https://doi.org/10.4102/curationis.v39i1.1558.

Rudman, A., & Gustavsson, J. P. (2011). Early-career burnout among new graduate nurses: A prospective observational study of intra-individual change trajectories. *International Journal of Nursing Studies, 48*(3), 292–306.

Sale, J. E. M., Lohfeld, L. H., & Brazil, K. (2002). Revisiting the Quantitative-Qualitative Debate: Implications for Mixed-Methods Research. *Quality and Quantity, 36*, 43–53. https://doi.org/10.1023/A:1014301607592.

Seidman, A. (2005). Minority student retention: Resources for practitioners. (2005). In G. H. Gaither (Ed.), *Minority retention: What works*, 7–24.

Seidman, A. (2018). *Crossing the Finish Line: How to Retain and Graduate Your Students*. Lanham, MD: Rowman & Littlefield.

Shinebourne, P. (2011). The Theoretical Underpinnings of Interpretive Phenomenological Analysis (IPA). *Existential Analysis, 22*(1), 16–31.

Smith, J. A., Flowers, P., & Larkin, M. (2009). *Interpretive Phenomenological Analysis: Theory, Method and Research*. London: Sage Publications.

Smith, J. A., & Osborn, M. (2008). Interpretive Phenomenological Analysis. (2008). In J. A. Smith (Ed.), *Qualitative Psychology: A Practical Guide to Research Methods*. London: Sage Publications.

Stelzer, F., Richard's, M. M., Andres, M. L., Vernucci, S., & Introzzi, I. (2019). Cognitive and maths-specific predictors of fraction conceptual knowledge. *Educational Psychology, 41*(2), 172–190. [Online]. https://doi.org/10.1080/01443410.2019.1693508. [Accessed 6 November 2023].

Taylor, J., Marland, G., Whitford, H., Carson, M., & Leece, R. (2022). Isolation and Marginalization: Exploring Attrition of Men in Preregistration Nursing Programs. *Journal of Nursing Education, 61*(4), 179–186. [Online]. https://doi.org/10.3928/01484834-20220209-02.

Tufano, V. C., Summers, E. J., & Covington, B. (2023). Motivators for nurse educators to persist in their profession: A phenomenological research study. *Nurse Education Today, 123*, 195725. [Online]. https://doi.org/10.1016/j.nedt.2023.105725.

University of Bolton (2018) *Data Protection Policy* [Online], Available from: https://www.bolton.ac.uk/assets/Uploads/Data-Protection-Policy-2018.pdf. Accessed June 2023.

University of Bolton (2023) *Research & Teaching Ethics Framework* [Online], Available from: https://www.bolton.ac.uk/join-us/research-programmes/research-policies-and-documents/research-ethics-framework. Accessed June 2023.

Urwin, S., Stanley, R., Jones, M., Gallagher, A., Wainwright, P., & Perkins, A. (2010). Understanding student nurse attrition: Learning from the literature. *Nurse Education Today, 30*(2), 202–207. [Online]. https://doi.org/10.1016/j.nedt.2009.07.014.

Weeks, K. W., Lyne, P., & Torrance, C. (2000). Written drug dosage errors made by students: the threat to clinical effectiveness and the need for a new approach. *Clinical Effectiveness in Nursing, 4*(1), 20–29. [Online]. https://doi.org/10.1054/cein.2000.0101. [Accessed 6 November 2023].

Wray, J., Aspland, J., Barrett, D., & Gardiner, E. (2017). Factors affecting the programme completion of pre-registration nursing students through a three-year course: A retrospective cohort study. *Nurse Education in Practice, 24*, 14–20. [Online]. https://doi.org/10.1016/j.nepr.2017.03.002.

CHAPTER 4

Factors Contributing to Attrition

Amanda Costello

Introduction

Student attrition has multilayered challenges influenced by a range of academic, psychosocial, workplace, financial, economic, cultural, and gender-related factors. Academically, students may struggle with rigorous coursework, inadequate preparation, or a lack of support systems, leading to disengagement and eventual dropout. Psychosocial factors, including mental health struggles, lack of motivation, and inadequate social support, further contribute to attrition by a decrease in the students' sense of belonging and ability to persist in their studies. Workplace exposure such as a demanding job in addition to the students' programme of study can create conflicts between academic commitments and work obligations, making it difficult for students to balance both effectively.

Financial and economic considerations also play a significant role in student retention, as tuition costs, living expenses, and the need for employment often place substantial pressure on students. Those from low-income backgrounds may face greater difficulties in affording education, leading to increased dropout rates. Furthermore, cultural and gender issues can impact students' experiences, with certain societal expectations or biases discouraging individuals, especially women and marginalised groups, from pursuing higher education or completing their programmes. These intersecting factors highlight the complexity of student attrition and emphasise the need for comprehensive strategies to improve retention and academic success.

Academic Factors

Student attrition is a persistent challenge in higher education, influenced by various academic factors that hinder student persistence and success. One of the most significant contributors is inadequate academic preparation. Many students enter university without the necessary foundational knowledge, particularly in subjects such as mathematics and writing, making it difficult to meet academic expectations. Tinto (1993) argues that students who experience early academic difficulties are more likely to disengage and eventually drop out. This lack of preparedness is often linked to disparities in secondary education quality, disproportionately affecting students from underprivileged backgrounds (Astin, 1997).

Another key factor is the rigor of academic programmes. While academic challenges are essential for intellectual growth, excessive difficulty can overwhelm students, leading to frustration and attrition. According to Kuh et al. (2008), students who perceive coursework as excessively demanding, without adequate support mechanisms such as tutoring or mentoring, are at a higher risk of leaving their studies prematurely. Additionally, assessment methods that do not accommodate diverse learning styles contribute to student disengagement. When students struggle with rigid evaluation systems that prioritise standardised testing over practical and critical thinking skills, they may feel disillusioned and opt to discontinue their studies (Yorke & Longden, 2004).

The role of institutional support is also crucial in academic persistence. Universities that provide comprehensive academic resources, such as writing centres, remedial courses, and proactive academic advising, tend to have lower dropout rates (Tinto, 2012). Conversely, institutions with limited academic support services often see higher attrition, particularly among first-generation college students who may lack guidance on how to navigate university expectations (Pascarella & Terenzini, 2005). Furthermore, large class sizes and limited faculty interaction contribute to a sense of academic alienation. Studies suggest that students who engage in meaningful interactions with faculty members are more likely to persist in their studies (Chickering & Gamson, 1987). When students feel like mere numbers in an impersonal system, they may struggle to stay motivated, thereby increasing their likelihood of dropping out.

Another academic factor leading to attrition is ineffective academic advising. Poorly structured or impersonal advising systems can result in students selecting inappropriate courses, delaying their academic progress, or failing to meet degree requirements (Habley, 2004). Effective advising plays a crucial role in ensuring that students make informed decisions about their educational pathways. When universities fail to provide accessible and personalised academic advising, students may become frustrated and opt to leave their programmes.

In conclusion, academic factors significantly contribute to student attrition, particularly in cases where institutions fail to provide adequate preparation, support, and guidance. A combination of rigorous academic expectations, insufficient institutional resources, large class sizes, and inadequate advising can create a challenging environment that discourages student persistence. To reduce attrition rates, higher education institutions must implement comprehensive academic support services, promote faculty–student engagement, and adopt flexible assessment methods that cater to diverse learning styles.

Psychosocial Factors

Attrition, defined as the gradual reduction in workforce numbers due to resignations, retirements, and other factors, is a pressing issue in many organisations. Various psychosocial factors contribute to attrition, encompassing workplace stress, job satisfaction, organisational culture, work–life balance, and social support. Understanding these factors can aid in developing effective retention strategies and improving employee well-being. This chapter explores the key psychosocial contributors to attrition, supported by academic references and relevant quotations.

WORKPLACE STRESS

Workplace stress is one of the most significant psychosocial contributors to attrition. Stress arises when job demands exceed an employee's capacity to cope, leading to burnout, disengagement, and eventual turnover. According to Schaufeli and Bakker (2004, p. 45), 'burnout is a persistent, negative work-related state of mind characterised by exhaustion, cynicism, and reduced professional efficacy'. High-stress environments, lack of autonomy, and excessive workload contribute to increased attrition rates.

JOB SATISFACTION AND MOTIVATION

Job satisfaction is a major predictor of attrition. Employees who find their work fulfilling and meaningful are more likely to stay, whereas those who experience dissatisfaction often seek other opportunities. The two-factor theory of Herzberg (1959) identifies job satisfaction as being influenced by intrinsic factors such as recognition, achievement, and responsibility. Conversely, hygiene factors, including poor working conditions and inadequate salary, contribute to dissatisfaction and eventual attrition. As Locke (1976, p. 23) posits, 'job satisfaction results from the perception that one's job fulfils or allows the fulfilment of one's important job values'.

ORGANISATIONAL CULTURE

A toxic or unsupportive organisational culture significantly contributes to attrition. When employees feel undervalued, experience discrimination, or perceive an absence of growth opportunities, they are more likely to leave. Research by Schein (2010, p. 82), highlights that 'organisational culture is a pattern of shared basic assumptions learned by a group as it solved its problems of external adaptation and internal integration'. A positive and inclusive work culture fosters commitment, whereas a negative culture leads to disengagement and high turnover rates.

WORK–LIFE BALANCE

Work–life balance is another critical factor influencing attrition. Employees may struggle to manage work demands alongside personal responsibilities, leading to stress and dissatisfaction. According to Greenhaus and Beutell, (1985, p. 12) 'work-family conflict occurs when role pressures from the work and family domains are mutually incompatible, making participation in both roles more difficult'. Organisations that fail to offer flexible work arrangements, remote work options, or paid leave policies see higher attrition rates.

LACK OF CAREER GROWTH OPPORTUNITIES

Career growth and development opportunities play a crucial role in employee retention. When employees perceive stagnation in their careers, they often seek better prospects elsewhere. According to Tansky and Cohen (2001, p. 13), 'career development opportunities and organisational support for learning are key to retaining skilled employees'. Lack of promotions, inadequate training programmes, and limited upward mobility contribute to attrition.

SOCIAL SUPPORT AND WORKPLACE RELATIONSHIPS

Workplace relationships and social support systems impact an employee's decision to stay or leave an organisation. Strong bonds with colleagues and supportive supervisors enhance job satisfaction and commitment. Conversely, workplace conflicts, lack of mentorship, and unsupportive leadership contribute to higher turnover. According to House (1981, p. 32) 'social support in the workplace acts as a buffer against job stress and enhances employee well-being'.

EMPLOYEE RECOGNITION AND REWARDS

A lack of recognition and rewards can demotivate employees, leading to increased attrition. Employees who feel that their efforts are not acknowledged often experience reduced commitment and morale. According to Deci and Ryan (1985, p. 35), 'intrinsic motivation thrives in environments where employees feel competent and autonomous'. Organisations that implement recognition programmes and provide fair compensation experience lower attrition rates.

PSYCHOLOGICAL CONTRACT BREACH

A psychological contract refers to the unwritten expectations between employees and employers. When employees perceive a breach in this contract such as unfulfilled promises regarding promotions, salary increases, or job security, it results in mistrust and disengagement. Rousseau (1995, p. 16) explains that 'psychological contract breaches lead to reduced job satisfaction, organisational commitment, and increased turnover intentions'.

COPING STRATEGIES AND ORGANISATIONAL INTERVENTIONS

To mitigate attrition, organisations must implement effective coping strategies and interventions. Providing employee assistance programmes (EAPs), fostering a supportive culture, and enhancing job design can significantly improve retention. Research by Allen et al. (2003) suggests that 'supportive HR [human resource] practices, including training, career development, and work-life balance initiatives, are crucial in reducing employee turnover.'

CONCLUSION

Attrition is a multilayered issue influenced by numerous psychosocial factors, including workplace stress, job satisfaction, organisational culture, work–life balance, career growth opportunities, social support, recognition, and psychological contract breaches. By addressing these factors through effective organisational policies and practices, companies can improve employee retention and create a more engaged workforce.

Workplace Exposure

Workplace attrition, particularly with respect to workplace exposure, is a multilayered issue that impacts organisations across industries. The concept of workplace exposure encompasses various elements, including environmental factors, job demands, stressors, and organisational culture, all of which contribute to an employee's decision to leave an organisation. Understanding these factors is crucial for businesses aiming to reduce turnover and retain top talent.

One of the primary factors influencing attrition is job stress. Workplace stress, resulting from excessive job demands, role ambiguity, and high work pressure, significantly contributes to employee turnover. Research indicates that chronic stress in the workplace not only affects an individual's physical and mental health but also leads to job dissatisfaction and eventual resignation (Cooper & Quick, 2017). A study by Bakker and Demerouti (2018) highlights that high job demands coupled with low job resources create burnout, which is a leading cause of attrition.

Toxic workplace environments also play a significant role in employee attrition. Exposure to workplace bullying, harassment, discrimination, or poor leadership can lead to job dissatisfaction and an employee's desire to exit an organisation. According to Einarsen et al. (2016), workplace bullying is a pervasive issue that results in psychological distress and decreased job commitment. Employees subjected to persistent negative behaviours from colleagues or supervisors often feel undervalued and unsupported, leading them to seek employment elsewhere.

Another key factor contributing to attrition is inadequate compensation and benefits. Employees exposed to financial stress due to low wages, lack of benefits, or unfair pay structures are more likely to leave in search of better opportunities. As per the equity theory of motivation, individuals compare their input-to-output ratio with that of their peers and feel dissatisfied if they perceive an imbalance (Adams, 1965). Empirical studies confirm that inadequate remuneration is a major driver of turnover, particularly in competitive job markets (Hausknecht et al., 2009).

Work–life balance is another crucial factor in workplace exposure that influences attrition. Employees who face excessive workloads, long hours, and unrealistic expectations often experience burnout and dissatisfaction. The work–family conflict theory suggests that an imbalance between work and personal life increases stress and decreases job commitment (Greenhaus & Beutell, 1985). Organisations that fail to provide flexible work arrangements or support employees' personal lives often witness high attrition rates (Kossek et al., 2011).

Leadership and managerial support are instrumental in employee retention. Employees who lack support from their supervisors often feel disengaged and unappreciated. Transformational leadership, which emphasises motivation, support, and personal development, has been shown to enhance job satisfaction and reduce turnover (Bass & Riggio, 2006). Conversely, autocratic or unsupportive leadership styles contribute to workplace dissatisfaction, fostering an environment where employees feel undervalued and unrecognised.

Career development opportunities are also essential in determining an employee's tenure within an organisation. Employees who perceive limited growth potential or lack professional development opportunities are more likely to leave. According to the human capital theory, employees invest in skills and education to increase their market value, and when organisations fail to support career advancement, employees seek opportunities elsewhere (Becker, 1964). Research supports the notion that companies with strong training and development programmes experience lower attrition rates.

Workplace safety and health concerns contribute to attrition, particularly in high-risk industries. Employees exposed to unsafe working conditions, physical hazards, or psychological stress due to workplace violence are more likely to leave their jobs. Occupational stress theory posits that prolonged exposure to workplace hazards leads to psychological strain, increasing the likelihood of turnover. Studies suggest that organizations prioritising employee health and safety have lower attrition rates, as employees feel more secure and valued in such environments (Cooper & Cartwright, 1994).

Organisational culture significantly influences employee retention. A toxic work culture characterised by poor communication, lack of transparency, and resistance to change leads to disengagement and turnover. Schein (2010) posits that organisational culture shapes employees' perceptions, attitudes, and behaviours, thereby affecting their commitment to the company. Companies that cultivate a positive, inclusive, and ethical work environment tend to retain employees for longer durations (Cameron & Quinn, 2011).

Technological changes and job automation also contribute to attrition, as employees exposed to rapid technological advancements may feel insecure about their job stability. The job-demand-control-support model suggests that employees who perceive a lack of control over their work environment are more likely to experience job dissatisfaction and seek alternative employment (Karasek, 1979). To mitigate this risk, organisations should invest in continuous learning and reskilling initiatives to help employees adapt to technological changes (Brynjolfsson & McAfee, 2014).

Finally, geographical factors and commuting stress contribute to attrition. Employees who experience long commute times or work in locations with limited accessibility often find it challenging to maintain job satisfaction. Companies offering remote work options or relocation assistance tend to mitigate this issue and enhance employee retention.

In conclusion, workplace exposure encompasses a variety of factors that influence attrition, including job stress, toxic work environments, inadequate compensation, work–life balance, leadership, career development opportunities, workplace safety, organisational culture, technological changes, and commuting stress. Organisations aiming to reduce turnover should implement policies that promote employee well-being, provide competitive compensation, foster supportive leadership, and create a positive work culture. By addressing these factors, businesses can enhance employee retention, boost productivity, and maintain a competitive advantage in the industry.

Financial and Economic Considerations

Employee attrition is a complex issue that organisations face globally, influenced by various financial and economic factors. Understanding these influences is crucial for companies seeking to mitigate turnover and retain talent. High attrition rates can lead to increased costs, reduced productivity, and loss of institutional knowledge, all of which can impact an organisation's long-term sustainability (Gong et al., 2018). This discussion critically examines the financial and economic aspects that need to be considered when analysing attrition, supported by references and quotations from scholars and experts.

One of the primary financial considerations in attrition is the cost associated with employee turnover. According to Cascio (2019), turnover costs include direct expenses such as recruitment, hiring, and training as well as indirect costs like lost productivity and decreased morale among remaining employees. "Replacing an employee can cost anywhere between 50% [and] 200% of their annual salary," according to Cascio (2019, p. 112), highlighting the financial burden that organisations face when employees leave. Given these costs, firms must develop retention strategies to minimise frequent exits and ensure financial stability.

Another financial aspect influencing attrition is compensation and benefits. Studies indicate that inadequate salaries, lack of bonuses, and insufficient benefits packages contribute significantly to employee dissatisfaction and eventual departure (Herzberg, 2003). Compensation plays a critical role in motivating employees, and when wages do not align with industry standards, workers may seek better-paying opportunities elsewhere. Thus organisations must ensure competitive compensation structures to retain talent.

Economic conditions also play a crucial role in employee attrition. During periods of economic downturns, attrition rates may decline as job opportunities become scarce. Conversely, during economic booms, employees may have more employment options, leading to higher turnover rates. For instance, the labour market trends in the aftermath of the COVID-19 pandemic demonstrated a phenomenon known as the Great Resignation, where employees left their jobs in pursuit of better work conditions, flexibility, and higher salaries (Klotz, 2021). Economic growth leads to increased job mobility, making it imperative for organisations to create attractive work environments to retain employees.

Job security is another economic factor that influences attrition. Employees in industries prone to layoffs, such as manufacturing or technology, often experience job insecurity, which may lead them to voluntarily exit before facing termination

(Berglund & Furåker, 2020). Research suggests that "job insecurity is one of the most significant predictors of voluntary turnover, as employees seek stability in uncertain economic conditions." Hence, organisations must foster a sense of job stability by ensuring transparent communication about company performance and future prospects.

Workplace conditions and career development opportunities are also important financial and economic factors impacting attrition. Lack of career advancement opportunities often leads employees to seek alternative employment where professional growth is possible. Companies that fail to provide skill development and upward mobility may experience higher turnover rates as workers prioritise career enhancement over job stability.

Inflation and cost-of-living adjustments also contribute to attrition. Employees working in regions with high living costs may feel financially strained if their wages do not increase accordingly. 'Workers tend to migrate towards organisations and locations that offer better financial sustainability in relation to living expenses' (Blau & Kahn, 2020, p. 657). Companies operating in high-cost areas must consider cost-of-living adjustments and housing benefits to retain their workforce.

The psychological contract between employees and employers plays a significant role in attrition as well. When employees perceive that their employer has failed to meet implicit agreements regarding pay raises, promotions, or job security, they may become disengaged and seek employment elsewhere. To prevent attrition, organisations must manage expectations transparently and fulfil commitments to their employees.

Work–life balance and job flexibility have become increasingly relevant in discussions of attrition, particularly in the postpandemic era. Employees now prioritise remote work options, flexible schedules, and work environments that support mental health and well-being. 'Organisations that fail to adapt to changing work-life expectations risk losing employees to competitors who offer greater flexibility' (Allen et al., 2021, p. 345). Companies that rigidly adhere to traditional work structures without accommodating modern work preferences may see higher attrition rates.

Cultural and generational shifts also influence attrition, with younger workers valuing different aspects of employment compared to previous generations. Millennials and Generation Z employees often seek purpose-driven work, rapid career progression, and workplace environments that align with their values. "Traditional retention strategies may not be effective for younger generations who prioritise experiences, learning opportunities, and corporate social responsibility." Organisations must therefore adjust their retention strategies to align with the evolving expectations of the modern workforce.

Employer branding and organisational reputation further impact attrition rates. Companies with strong employer brands attract and retain employees more effectively than those with negative reputations. 'Employees want to be associated with organisations that uphold strong values, provide development opportunities, and treat their workforce fairly' (Backhaus & Tikoo, 2004, p. 507). A company perceived as having a toxic work culture or unethical practices may struggle with high turnover rates as employees seek organisations with better reputations.

Lastly, leadership and management styles significantly affect attrition. Poor leadership, lack of recognition, and ineffective management practices contribute to employee dissatisfaction. Research suggests that "employees do not leave jobs; they leave managers." Effective leaders who provide mentorship, support, and constructive feedback create environments where employees feel valued and are less likely to leave.

In conclusion, financial and economic factors play a crucial role in determining attrition rates within organisations. High turnover costs, inadequate compensation, economic conditions, job security concerns, lack of career growth, inflation, work–life balance, generational differences, employer branding, and leadership quality all contribute to an employee's decision to stay or leave. Organisations that proactively address these factors through competitive compensation, strong leadership, transparent communication, and a positive workplace culture can reduce attrition and foster long-term employee engagement.

Cultural and Gender Issues

Attrition, defined as the gradual reduction of a workforce through voluntary or involuntary departures, poses significant challenges for organisations aiming to maintain a stable and skilled employee base. Cultural and gender-related factors play pivotal roles in influencing attrition rates, often intertwining to create complex dynamics that affect employee retention.

Organisational culture encompasses the shared values, beliefs, and practices that shape the work environment. A culture that lacks inclusivity or perpetuates gender biases can lead to increased turnover, particularly among underrepresented groups. For instance, a survey highlighted that 60% of women who exited the workforce attributed their departure to unfavourable organisational culture, citing issues such as patriarchal team dynamics and low inclusivity (Sarkar, 2020). Such environments can foster feelings of isolation and undervaluation among female employees, prompting them to seek opportunities elsewhere.

Gender discrimination within the workplace significantly impacts turnover intentions. Research indicates that perceived gender discrimination correlates with decreased career satisfaction, which in turn increases the likelihood of employees considering resignation (Murat-Eminoğlu, 2021). This relationship describes the importance of equitable treatment and opportunities for all employees, regardless of gender.

The concept of the 'leaky pipeline' is particularly prevalent in STEM (Science, Technology, Engineering, and Mathematics) fields, where women are underrepresented. Despite entering these fields, many women leave due to obstacles such as gender bias and unequal promotion opportunities. A report by Sangeeta (2023) emphasises that investing in leadership development programmes tailored to address these challenges can mitigate gender-based attrition by empowering managers to create supportive work environments.

Numerical minority status also plays a crucial role in attrition rates. A study examining women's attrition from male-dominated workplaces in Norway found that as the percentage of male employees increased, so did the likelihood of women leaving these environments (Madsen et al., 2023). This trend was consistent across various occupational classes, suggesting that being in the minority can lead to heightened feelings of isolation and discomfort, driving higher turnover rates among women.

Stereotypes and cultural perceptions further exacerbate gender disparities in employment. Traditional views often undervalue women's contributions, leading to biases in hiring, promotion, and compensation. Such stereotypes can result in women receiving lower wages and limited growth opportunities, reinforcing a cycle of attrition as they seek more equitable workplaces (Fitzsimmons et al., 2014).

High attrition rates can also negatively impact workplace culture, creating a vicious cycle where a deteriorating culture leads to further turnover. A survey revealed that 63% of UK businesses experienced cultural decline due to high staff attrition, with issues such as decreased employee engagement and the development of toxic work environments being reported (Moss, 2022). This highlights the interconnectedness of culture and retention, where challenges in one area can significantly affect the other.

To address these issues, organisations must implement comprehensive strategies that promote inclusivity and equity. This includes developing leadership programmes that sensitise managers to gender biases, fostering a culture that values diversity, and ensuring transparent career progression paths. By proactively addressing cultural and gender-related factors, organisations can enhance employee satisfaction and reduce attrition rates.

In conclusion, cultural and gender issues are deeply intertwined with employee attrition. Organisations that fail to recognise and address these factors risk perpetuating cycles of turnover that can undermine their stability and growth. Conversely, those that actively cultivate inclusive and equitable cultures are better positioned to retain talent and foster long-term success.

References

Adams, J. S. (1965). Inequity in social exchange. *Advances in Experimental Social Psychology, 2*, 267–299.

Allen, D. G., Shore, L. M., & Griffeth, R. W. (2003). The role of perceived organizational support and supportive human resource practices in the turnover process. *Journal of Management, 29*(1), 99–118.

Allen, T. D., Cho, E., & Meier, L. L. (2021). Work–family boundary dynamics. *Annual Review of Organizational Psychology and Organizational Behavior, 8*, 345–367.

Astin, A. W. (1997). *What matters in college? Four critical years revisited.* Jossey-Bass.

Backhaus, K., & Tikoo, S. (2004). Conceptualizing and researching employer branding. *Career Development International, 9*(5), 501–517.

Bakker, A. B., & Demerouti, E. (2018). Burnout and job performance: The moderating role of selection, optimization, and compensation strategies. *Journal of Occupational Health Psychology, 23*(1), 28–40.

Bass, B. M., & Riggio, R. E. (2006). *Transformational leadership*. Psychology Press.

Becker, G. S. (1964). *Human capital: A theoretical and empirical analysis, with special reference to education*. University of Chicago Press.

Berglund, T., & Furåker, B. (2020). Job insecurity and economic uncertainty: A theoretical perspective. *Work, Employment and Society, 34*(4), 635–652.

Blau, F. D., & Kahn, L. M. (2020). The gender wage gap: Extent, trends, and explanations. *Journal of Economic Literature, 58*(3), 657–702.

Brynjolfsson, E., & McAfee, A. (2014). *The second machine age: Work, progress, and prosperity in a time of brilliant technologies*. W. W. Norton & Company.

Cameron, K. S., & Quinn, R. E. (2011). *Diagnosing and changing organizational culture: Based on the competing values framework*. John Wiley & Sons.

Cascio, W. F. (2019). *Managing human resources*. McGraw-Hill Education.

Chickering, A. W., & Gamson, Z. F. (1987). Seven principles for good practice in undergraduate education. *AAHE Bulletin, 39*(7), 3–7.

Cooper, C. L., & Cartwright, S. (1994). Healthy mind; healthy organization—A proactive approach to occupational stress. *Human Relations, 47*(4), 455–471.

Cooper, C. L., & Quick, J. C. (2017). *The handbook of stress and health: A guide to research and practice*. John Wiley & Sons.

Deci, E. L., & Ryan, R. M. (1985). *Intrinsic motivation and self-determination in human behavior*. Springer Science & Business Media.

Einarsen, S., Hoel, H., Zapf, D., & Cooper, C. L. (2016). *Bullying and harassment in the workplace: Developments in theory, research, and practice*. CRC Press.

Fitzsimmons, T. W., Callan, V. J., & Paulsen, N. (2014). Gender disparity in employment: Stereotypes and cultural perceptions. *Journal of Management & Organization, 20*(4), 467–482.

Gong, Y., Wang, M., Huang, J. C., & Cheung, S. Y. (2018). Toward a goal-setting perspective on employee turnover. *Journal of Management, 44*(5), 1939–1967.

Gotara. (2023). The impact of leadership development on gender-based attrition. Retrieved from https://www.gotara.com/the-impact-of-leadership-development-on-gender-based-attrition/.

Greenhaus, J. H., & Beutell, N. J. (1985). Sources of conflict between work and family roles. *Academy of Management Review, 10*(1), 76–88.

Habley, W. R. (2004). The status of academic advising: Findings from the ACT sixth national survey. *National Academic Advising Association Journal, 24*(1-2), 5–19.

Hausknecht, J. P., Trevor, C. O., & Howard, M. J. (2009). Unit-level voluntary turnover rates and customer service quality: Implications of group cohesion and subgroup differences. *Journal of Applied Psychology, 94*(4), 1068–1075.

Herzberg, F. (1959). *The motivation to work*. John Wiley & Sons.

Herzberg, F. (2003). *One more time: How do you motivate employees? Harvard Business Review Press.*

House, J. S. (1981). *Work stress and social support*. Addison-Wesley.

Karasek, R. A. (1979). Job demands, job decision latitude, and mental strain: Implications for job redesign. *Administrative Science Quarterly, 24*(2), 285–308.

Klotz, A. (2021). The Great Resignation: Why employees are quitting in record numbers. *Harvard Business Review.*

Kossek, E. E., Pichler, S., Bodner, T., & Hammer, L. B. (2011). Workplace social support and work-family conflict: A meta-analysis clarifying the influence of general and work-family-specific supervisor and organisational support. *Personnel Psychology, 64*(2), 289–313.

Kuh, G. D., Kinzie, J., Buckley, J. A., Bridges, B. K., & Hayek, J. C. (2008). *Piecing together the student success puzzle: Research, propositions, and recommendations*. ASHE Higher Education Report.

Locke, E. A. (1976). The nature and causes of job satisfaction. In M. D. Dunnette (Ed.), *Handbook of industrial and organisational psychology* (pp. 1297–1349). Rand McNally.

Madsen, A.Å., Brekke, I., & Fekjær, S. B. (2023). Women's attrition from male-dominated workplaces in Norway: The importance of numerical minority status, motherhood, and class. *Work, Employment and Society, 37*(1), 123–142.

Moss, R. (2022). Two thirds say high attrition is damaging workplace culture. *Personnel Today*. Retrieved from https://www.personneltoday.com/hr/attrition-workplace-culture-damaging/.

Murat-Eminoğlu, G. (2021). Perceived gender discrimination and turnover intention: The mediating role of career satisfaction. *European Proceedings of Social and Behavioural Sciences, 122*, 67–74.

Pascarella, E. T., & Terenzini, P. T. (2005). *How college affects students: A third decade of research*. Jossey-Bass.

Rousseau, D. M. (1995). *Psychological contracts in organizations: Understanding written and unwritten agreements*. Sage Publications.

Sarkar, B. (2020). Six in 10 women, who drop out of the workforce, blame organisational culture at previous workplace. *The Economic Times*. Retrieved from https://economictimes.indiatimes.com/magazines/panache/six-in-10-women-who-drop-out-of-the-workforce-blame-organisational-culture-at-previous-workplace/articleshow/79833336.cms. Accessed June 2025.

Schein, E. H. (2010). *Organisational culture and leadership*. John Wiley & Sons.

Schaufeli, W. B., & Bakker, A. B. (2004). Job demands, job resources, and their relationship with burnout and engagement: A multi-sample study. *Journal of Organisational Behaviour, 25*(3), 293–315.

Tansky, J. W., & Cohen, D. J. (2001). The relationship between organizational support, employee development, and organisational commitment: An empirical study. *Human Resource Development Quarterly, 12*(3), 285–300.

Tinto, V. (1993). *Leaving college: Rethinking the causes and cures of student attrition*. University of Chicago Press.

Tinto, V. (2012). *Completing college: Rethinking institutional action*. University of Chicago Press.

Yorke, M., & Longden, B. (2004). *Retention and student success in higher education*. McGraw-Hill Education.

CHAPTER 5

Personal Idiosyncratic Reasons for Leaving an Undergraduate Nursing Course

Amanda Costello

Introduction

The decision to leave an undergraduate nursing programme is often complex and deeply personal. While institutional factors such as academic challenges, financial constraints, and workload pressures are commonly discussed, personal idiosyncratic reasons unique to each individual also play a significant role. These reasons may stem from changes in personal interests, unexpected life circumstances, mental and emotional well-being, or a reevaluation of long-term career aspirations. Understanding these personal motivations can provide valuable insights into student retention, well-being, and the broader implications for nursing education. This chapter explores the diverse and individualised reasons students may choose to discontinue their nursing studies, highlighting the importance of personal fulfilment, adaptability, and institutional support in academic persistence.

NHS England Research Results and Findings

INTRODUCTION TO FINDINGS

The research findings were based on seven superordinate themes that emerged from the Interpretative Phenomenological Analysis (IPA) process: (1) Barriers to learner engagement, (2) Additional support, (3) Intervention and engagement, (4) Successful learning, (5) Sense of self, (6) Learner at risk beliefs, and (7) Relationship beliefs and practice. These themes, along with their accompanying subordinate themes, are explored with the aim of providing the reader with a rich account of the researchers of participants' lived experiences. The researchers then discuss the findings of this NHS England research project in light of extant literature and theory concerned with agency, structure, and reflexivity.

PARTICIPANTS' DEMOGRAPHIC CHARACTERISTICS

In-depth, semistructured interviews were conducted with 20 undergraduate nurses between February and May 2023. None of the participants opted for a telephone interview; one student was interviewed using Zoom, and the remaining students had face-to-face interviews. The participants who took part in this study were between 18 and 55 years of age at the time of interview. All participants were undergraduate nurses in a direct entry programme or apprenticeship programme at the University of Bolton and the satellite Higher Education Institute at Bradford and Devon.

THEMES AND ANALYTIC COMMENTARY

The findings of this NHS England research project show how the participants' experience of undergraduate nursing has been shaped by structure and agency. However, examination of the data revealed a large degree of heterogeneity between participants; each participant described mediating and making sense of structural forces and their agentic capacity to act in a different way. The IPA of undergraduate nurses' accounts produced seven superordinate themes. These themes were labelled as follows: (1) Barriers to learner engagement, (2) Additional support, (3) Intervention and engagement, (4) Successful learning, (5) Sense of self, (6) Learner at risk beliefs, and (7) Relationship beliefs and practice.

Each of the themes details different aspects of undergraduate nurses' lived experiences and perceptions, using illustrative quotations to highlight the convergences and divergences among participants.

Superordinate Theme (1): Barriers to Learner Engagement

The first superordinate theme, 'Barriers to learner engagement', relates to the challenges and restrictions that the researchers' participants reported having to actively negotiate during their undergraduate nursing programme. The data collected under this theme demonstrate how the professional and home lives of the participants intertwine with a cause and effect. This superordinate theme comprises two subordinate themes: (1) Assessment issues and family constraints and (2) Language, attendance, and access.

ASSESSMENT ISSUES AND FAMILY CONSTRAINTS

One of the ways in which the researchers' participants appeared to have made sense of their experience of assessment was to track their own progress in relation to failed modules due to personal events and circumstances. There were eight mothers in the researchers' sample, and all eight spoke about having to consciously strike a balance between the multiple and competing responsibilities of motherhood, and how home responsibilities affected their learning during assessment times. Each participant had a varied experience of assessment learning outcomes and their struggle with family life and childcare.

One of the participants in the sample, Participant N, recalled her recent experience of assessment and explained she had a learning contract and required additional support and differentiation of the expected learning outcomes. Participant N described her anxiety and confusion of the assessment processes in her undergraduate nursing programme, stating, 'I don't quite understand what I have to do when I am given an assessment to complete' (N, page 1, line 4).

Participant N explained that she did not always understand the written terms in examination questions or assessment papers. She started to demonstrate low self-esteem and elements of lack of motivation. 'I struggle to answer questions in exams and I don't understand the context. I try to read more, but become frustrated due to my lack of knowledge and understanding' (N, page 1, line 5).

Participant N was describing how she felt about assessment and her lack of knowledge and understanding; she had other complex issues of not being able to study to achieve her nursing goals. She explained, 'Sometimes my children and family problems have a big impact on my learning' (N, page 1, lines 7–8).

A situation is exacerbated when there are young children to look after and added wider family issues. Participant N highlighted a sense of pride that she was able to handle her children singlehandedly and without a partner to support her. She also highlighted that her nursing studies were suffering, and if she understood her assessment expectation, it would not be as difficult and she would not miss time away from university.

This raises the question regarding learning contracts and additional support required for learners. Participant N clearly states that additional stresses and strains of family life have a 'big impact on my learning' (N, page 1, line 8).

Participant M, like Participant N, explained that assessment was difficult, as she had many problems with assessment not being explained clearly. 'I find it difficult to manage my time and I then start to lack confidence' (M, page 1, line 3). In Participant M's interview the researcher recovered many differing elements to Participant M's level of confidence and self-esteem. She explained to the researcher, 'Some learners are shy, and they probably don't like to engage too much and this leads to problems during assessments' (M, page 1, line 4). Participant M went on to state: 'Lack of engagement stops you learning' (M, page 1, line 5). 'I think this is why some students stop engaging with the programme' (M, page 1, line 6). 'I sit at the back in lectures because I am shy—but I do want to engage' (M, page 1, line 13).

Participant M was explicit when she described her barriers to learning, and these being undetected by university staff can in turn lead to learner attrition.

Participant I resonated with the other two learners and added that 'being an adult student can lead to low levels of confidence and the fear of failing a module' (I, page 1, lines 2–3).

Participant A explained that much of her hindrance to achieving in assessment is that she is 'unable to concentrate at home. My mum has so many children and I am unable to concentrate; she then wants me to look after the younger children whilst she does other stuff. I have already failed several modules and I am at risk of failing my course. I can't afford to move out of the family home' (A, page 1, lines 6–8).

Two divergent and conflicting discourses emerge from these extracts: learning intervention and identification of learning needs within nursing cohorts. These discourses are reinforced by Participant Q, who stated, 'I am dyslexic and also have

ADHD – I have read and write software which is on my computer and I also have extra time for my assessments and exams' (Q, page 1, line 3).

Other participants interviewed chimed the statements of each other, and the researchers were again clear about their individual learning struggles.

Participant R said, 'It is difficult not being able to access things that will improve my learning capacity for the future. For example, if I can access electronic resources and the library, I don't get frustrated; frustration does hinder my learning' (R, page 1, lines 6–8).

Participant E explained her barrier to assessment learning, stating, 'I think it's not understanding why you are learning things. I don't really understand why we are learning about global health; I feel we need to learn regionally in nursing. Our learning needs to be linked to the ward or in a hospital/community environment, otherwise it isn't as interesting. Most people are engaged in clinical skills because we know this is what we are going to need' (E, page 1, lines 5–15).

A final thought on assessment from Participant H: 'The key assessment barrier is students not having enough support from the school and lecturers having too high a workload on their time management; this affects how they explain assessment and our learning' (H, page 1, lines 3–5).

In summary, the subordinate theme 'Assessment issues and family constraints' represents the individual's ongoing and conscious negotiation within their undergraduate nursing studies and family responsibilities. It reveals a great deal of diversity in the ways in which the individual women in this study perceived and managed their nursing studies with childcare responsibilities. While some of the women reported feeling constrained by the (actual or potential) expectation to study and pass their assessments and exams and care for their families, others described feeling frustrated due to lack of support and heavy assessment workloads. A key feature in the participants' interviews was how self-esteem and confidence can be eroded during assessment and how these aspects affect assessment success and can lead to failed modules and placements.

LANGUAGE, ATTENDANCE, AND ACCESS

The subordinate theme 'Language, attendance, and access' allowed participants to discuss how English not being their first language affected learning and assessment success. There were six participants in this interview sample.

Each of the participants was able to discuss the difficulties of having to navigate the English language in the university's assessment protocols, including prepared resources for assessment and examination. Participant S was able to state that her learning was affected by her language barrier: 'The language barrier does affect me, but I know it also affects other students' (S, page 1, line 3).

Participant L was able to mirror Participant S's language barrier concerns. 'I am a second-year student nurse, and English is not my first language; I need support from the university and the library. I feel that sometimes people may laugh at me because of my accent, so it does stop me asking questions in the class' (L, page 1, line 5).

Participant L's description demonstrates how the learner's self-esteem and confidence had been affected by her language, and there was evidence to suggest that the participant was seeking additional support from the university and the campus library to support her language development and understanding of learning resources. Participant L was able to explain the multiple issues that were affecting her overall learning success: 'I face barriers with children as a single parent and also have to face the family courts due to domestic violence and financial problems. I juggle everything and also use public transport which can be a further struggle due to rail strikes; all these issues have affected my learning and I have recently failed a module and an exam' (L, page 1, lines 10–12).

Participant G was explicit when discussing the linguistic challenges: 'Language barrier is a barrier to learning; we need people to speak in the right tone and pitch, so that we understand the English language clearly. I also face the difficulty of having a family, so that makes having responsibilities and learning difficult; everything becomes a challenge, I would say' (G, page 1, lines 2–6).

The testimonies given by learners are a concern, and it is clear from the learners' voices that many are finding their undergraduate nursing course difficult due to language, access, and the overall impact on their university and placement attendance.

Participant F's interview was emotional and at times difficult due to the participant's learning journey: 'I am sorry to say English is not my first language; I have barriers to my learning. I came from overseas. I was a qualified nurse back home—I have no family or friends here . . . so I have had to do all the research for everything on my own. It has been very difficult' (F, page 1, lines 4–11). The learner in this case was already describing an uphill struggle within the learning and was apologising for English not being her first language: 'Even though I have worked in healthcare in the past I need a clear path for learning' (F, page 1, line 14).

Additionally, Participant F was assessing her own learning needs at this point and was reaching out for additional support. 'My language barrier has been an issue. In the beginning, I had no access to college, university or open days. I had a lack of guidance and instruction – who should I contact? Where should I go?' (F, page 1, line 18).

Participant F's experiential learning journey is harrowing and difficult to hear; it is clear from the interview that the participant had felt isolated and unheard, with the additional fact of being qualified as a nurse in her home country. She wanted to be clear that the researcher understood her starting points in her difficult lived learning experience.

> *'I redid Level 2 Maths and English, passed my Socrative and became a Nursing Associate. I am now doing a top-up and in my third year; it has taken me ten years from scratch. When I sat my IELTS exam I found it very difficult—even accessing my scores was a nightmare. When I did get my score, I was told my qualification from overseas was too old . . . that's why I had to start again' (F, page 1, lines 26–32).*

The learning journey experienced by Participant F has demonstrated high levels of motivation and resilience; her sheer determination has led to Participant F's success at the end of the third year of learning.

Participant K was thankful for having been given the opportunity to have a voice: 'Thank you for giving me the opportunity to give my point of view and to tell you what stops me from learning . . . French is my first language; I am a single mum with three children and I commute a long way from my home to the university and my placements. Travelling for me is a big issue and it hinders my timekeeping and learning as I am too tired' (K, page 1, lines 2–6).

The preceding example gives evidence of the levels of difficulty that learners may face relating to language, access, and attendance. Participant K, who has a learning contract, went on to explain: 'It is sometimes difficult because being bilingual and Greek, it is sometimes difficult to understand words in English . . . I have found myself asking peers at the beginning of a lesson. I also end up doing my assignment twice in Greek and in English . . . I also live alone; finances are tight, I walk or use public transport – this can be difficult – despite this I am still here and doing my best' (K, page 1, lines 7–11).

In summary, the subordinate theme 'Language, access, and attendance' represents the participants' levels of motivation and resilience during their undergraduate nursing studies. The participants' lived experiences are unique to them as individuals and demonstrate a high level of grit and determination. There are many facets that learners have to navigate to become successful learners. The evidence gives the reader explicit information relating to the daily struggles experienced by the learner in terms of language, prior learning qualifications, access and attendance issues, and financial constraints. There are many divergences, and learners have relied on their own initiative and have strived to learn and find out information relating to their undergraduate nursing programme. A key feature in each participant's lived experience is their level of isolation and difficulty in accessing information for their learning purposes.

Superordinate Theme (2): Additional Support

The two superordinate theme, 'Additional support', is pertinent to learners for whom English is not their first language and those who have said that they experienced difficulty in accessing assessment materials and resources. Accessing the university creates issues for learners regarding childcare and financial constraints.

Learners identified literacy and numeracy as areas of learning where they needed the most support. This superordinate theme comprises four subordinate themes: (1) Assessment understanding, (2) Access to university and teaching and learning, (3) Literacy and numeracy, and (4) English not first language.

ASSESSMENT UNDERSTANDING

This subordinate theme drills down further into the understanding of assessment. In the interview sample, seven participants were able to discuss their understanding of assessment and how assessment practices affected their individual learning and success.

Participant U explained, 'I need support with exams and assessments; lecturers need to know what we may be struggling with in terms of our assessment. I didn't understand some of the questions in my last assessment; I honestly had to make a guess . . . it turned out to be a good guess in the end' (U, page 2, lines 10–18).

Participant J said, 'Some people speak out for help, whereas others are more cautious. I am dyslexic – I didn't learn or go to school in Africa. When I was twenty years old, I came to Britain and I learnt to read and write. Women were not supposed to educate themselves; this is why I love this country . . . I am now the first female in my family to go to university' (J, page 2, lines 31–38).

Both preceding participants had difficulty understanding assessments, and more support is required to ensure that each participant has success in their learning outcomes.

Participant P explained that support needed is twofold: 'We need ongoing support with assessment understanding and more targeted support from our personal tutors' (P, page 2, line 8).

Participant I went one step further and explained that 'a more tailored approach to aid assessment understanding is needed; I would like to be assessed on my weaknesses and I would find this helpful to improve my learning. I would also like to see more communication with my lecturers' (I, page 2, lines 7–10). It is clear to the researchers that learners are wanting further clarity on assessment understanding. Other learner examples are further highlighted next.

In Participant N's interview, the participant mentioned a learning contract and additional needs. 'Sometimes a short test at the end of a teaching session will help to gauge understanding . . . a question-and-answer session and raised hands . . . we need support, but it is not seen online or in the classroom face to face, only when we fail our assessments' (N, page 2, lines 11–14).

Participant S's interview outlined the importance of diagnostic assessments in areas of weakness: 'It was helpful to have a baseline assessment for my maths ability and to sit and pass the maths paper for my Medicine Management learning. It narrows it down to seeing what questions you see on the actual exam; it also alleviates any fear seeing a past paper and knowing that the maths equations are essential for patient safety' (S, page 2, lines 8–15).

Participant B said, 'I think it is good that we do a formative assessment before our final summative assessment. I feel proud that I have submitted my final summative assessment work' (B, page 2, lines 22–24).

In summary, the subordinate theme 'Assessment understanding' demonstrates the participants' thoughts and feelings about this theme; some participants are underconfident with the assessment processes and would like a clearer explanation of the expected learning outcomes in their nursing modules. Other learners have a learning contract in place and would benefit from intervention classes to support their learning goals. Divergences within the transcripts give rise to the importance of diagnostic assessments and baseline assessments in the learning of new concepts. Participants outlined the usefulness of formative assessment and how this process increased their individual knowledge and understanding. Learners were able to say how proud they felt after assessment achievement.

ACCESS TO UNIVERSITY AND TEACHING AND LEARNING

This subordinate theme addresses participants' access to university and their teaching and learning experiences. There were 12 participants in the sample: 2 participants were able to discuss access to university, and the remaining 10 participants discussed their individual experiences of teaching and learning.

Participant E said, 'I am happy to be learning at the university and feel lucky to be studying. I think we do well with our tutorials and as a group we work well together and support each other' (E, page 2, lines 17–19).

Participant G's interview was like that of Participant E: 'I am grateful to be learning at this university; I have tried hard with my studies to gain a place on the nursing course. I started my learning when I moved to England with my family' (G, page 2, lines 8–9).

The university has given both participants the opportunity to learn, and both are happy to be learning in a nurturing environment. Both participants have shown a level of resilience within their approach to their studies in a widening participation university, giving access to learning for all.

The 10 participants in the sample interviews had a variety of testimonies whereby they individually expressed their views on teaching and learning.

Participant K explained, 'In the early days, I had support from my personal tutor; I was experiencing difficulties with my English writing. I worked with my tutor slowly and she was able to teach me how to access my learning online and how to use Moodle; she even taught me how to use my email. I have received a lot of support from Leap Online and I have found Maths for Nurses helpful' (K, page 2, lines 8–10).

Participant L was able to talk about learning in the same vein: 'I have attended Leap Online sessions and the classes have helped me with academic writing for research and also writing tips' (L, page 2, lines 22–23).

The importance of support systems to enable students to thrive in their university journey cannot be overemphasised. It is clear from the transcripts that some students have already identified the support that is required for their studies.

Participant T said, 'I think I would ask the librarian for help and support finding books and journals. I am in the process of having my learning contract put in place' (T, page 2, lines 19–21). Participant Q is also aware and states, 'I do access additional support, which is very helpful; I have a learning contract in place' (Q, page 2, lines 24–25).

Participant C stated that 'some learners have learning contracts and will let their tutors know if they are struggling' (C, page 2, line 32).

The researchers have found that this is not the case for all learners. Participant R feels that at times she is unable to express to her tutor that she is facing difficulties with learning. 'Communication with students needs to increase; online learning is difficult as you are unable to ask questions and explain things that you don't understand' (R, page 2, lines 12–15).

Participant H said that she finds learning hard: 'I wish the lecturers would understand that at times learning is difficult. I need support in English and Maths as

English is not my first language; provision for additional support needs making for me now!' (H, page 2, lines 10–12.) This learner wants immediate support and feels frustrated and unsupported.

Participant A said, 'I have finally received my dyslexia assessment results and at last I have a laptop and individual support with my learning. I was ready to give up last month as I had failed yet another module' (A, page 2, lines 13–14).

Participant M liked the one-to-one tutor sessions and said, 'The sessions are good for my learning and understanding of the expected learning outcomes for my module' (M, page 2, line 19).

Participant O is aligned with Participant M: 'I receive additional support from the Hub and Student Services; it has helped a lot, and I am thankful' (O, page 2, line 17).

In summary, the subordinate theme 'Access to university and teaching and learning' demonstrates the participants' understanding of how to access the university for their teaching and learning. Some participants are underconfident with the teaching and learning processes and would like a clearer explanation of the expected learning outcomes in their nursing modules. Other learners have a learning contract in place and would benefit from intervention classes to support their learning goals. Participants in this sample have been able to express themselves clearly about their learning needs and are grateful to have finally received a dyslexia diagnosis and to have more support for their teaching and learning needs such as a laptop and individual support.

ENGLISH NOT FIRST LANGUAGE

This subordinate theme is addressed throughout the research. Two participants found their language to be a real barrier to their learning. Participant F would like more guidance to support her interpretation of the English language, both written and spoken. 'Learning materials need to be clear; it then makes the research clear. I also have applied many times for the nursing course and they haven't come back to me. I would say it has been the language barrier; now I am learning I try my best, but it is not always easy' (F, page 2, line 38).

Participant D stated, 'I need more money to survive the course. Working and learning is hard; at the beginning of the programme I struggled a lot; my tutor gave me help. Most of my struggles are financial and language difficulties. Sometimes the university doesn't offer enough support and I know lack of support also affects other learners; we don't feel part of the wider university' (D, page 2, line 31).

In summary, the subordinate themes 'Access to university and teaching and learning' and 'English not first language' both represent the participants' struggles with teaching and learning during their undergraduate nursing studies. The participants' lived experiences are difficult and allow the researchers to understand how learning affects undergraduate nurses and how the issues can lead to attrition. The language barriers and financial constraints feature heavily for some learners, as do learning disabilities and access to learning. Some divergences show learners to be accessing additional learning and to have a learning contract in place. The use of the university's additional support services has been appreciated by some learners but not all.

Superordinate Theme (3): Intervention and Engagement

The third superordinate theme, 'Intervention and engagement', relates to participants' view of how they learn and their individual engagement within the undergraduate nursing programme. Under this superordinate theme, learners were able to articulate their struggles both within the university and their home life. The data collected under this theme gave insights into the support that learners would like to receive and examples of what good learning looked like for them individually.

This superordinate theme gives rise to four subordinate themes: (1) Learner engagement, (2) Learning struggles, (3) Learner support, and (4) Success in learning.

LEARNER ENGAGEMENT

This subordinate theme has a focus of the engagement of learners. Four participants found engagement with the undergraduate nursing programme difficult and expressed their views relating to low self-esteem and low learning starting points. One participant has an undiagnosed learning need and unaddressed emotional and mental health issues including anxiety.

Participant J said that she had always wanted to be a nurse: 'I want to be a good nurse and have worked hard with my studies to gain a place on the nursing programme. I know that I have low starting points; that does make me feel even more anxious; I suffer with anxiety and my emotional mental health. I have recently been assessed for dyslexia – it has been difficult studying towards my assessments; I have failed some assessments' (J, page 2, lines 43–51).

Participant N explained, 'When you have a learning disability, it is difficult to prepare for learning; it is important that the lecturer has that awareness too' (N, page 2, line 20).

Another example given by Participant N was of interest to the researchers. 'The lecturer gave me support details for my learning – I contacted the support service suggested . . . I received no reply . . . I have disbelief in the service now – there was no active support group working. I failed my assessment . . . I felt so disappointed and just wanted to pack it all in' (N, page 2, lines 21–23).

Participant A has found engagement with online learning difficult, and this has led to her disengagement at times: 'I live in a household with children under four years of age; my mum has five children. Working online is just not an option – I am disturbed all the time. I would like face-to-face learning to keep me onboard; I am by nature and by my learning needs easily distracted' (A, page 2, lines 24–26).

Participant R backs up what Participant A stressed in her interview. 'I struggle to engage and need to be more proficient in my Medicine Management module. I find drug calculations hard and don't always understand the SI doses' (R, page 2, line 26).

In this sample of four participants' disengagement, mental health and well-being are a feature of learners being at risk of attrition. In intervention and engagement, addressing the academic challenges faced by learners is essential in mitigating attrition rates amongst undergraduate nurses.

In summary, the subordinate theme 'Learner engagement' has given learners the opportunity to express their views and worries about their own levels of engagement. The participants' representation has shown that some undergraduate nursing learners find the programme difficult and have explained in their individual interviews their concerns about their low starting points and how this has affected their self-esteem. One participant has an undiagnosed learning need and unaddressed emotional and mental health issues and anxiety. Another participant has additional needs and has recently been diagnosed with dyslexia. The participants discussed their learning issues and wanted to tell their lecturers that this was about their individual needs. Some learners want more understanding and would like to slow down the pace of learning to enable success in their learning. Learners express their views and add further divergences, such as their struggle with drug calculations and wanting more support to enable their 100% pass mark. Others find online learning extremely difficult, as they must navigate young children in the household under the age of 4 years and there is no quiet space, and the library pods and spaces are often all booked. Learners at the satellite sites have expressed that finding a learning space can be hard.

LEARNER STRUGGLES

This subordinate theme demonstrates the struggles felt by undergraduate nursing students. Six participants in the sample described their struggles with studies during the undergraduate nursing programme. Participant B demonstrated multiple struggles in her learning journey. 'I have suffered domestic violence and find myself in the family court. I am trying to do my studies and finances are tight. I haven't got the time to fight all these battles; my children and studies come first. A good nursing job will help me to feed and clothe my family . . . I am on my own and I feel very isolated, you know' (B, page 2, lines 26–30).

Participant I explained that she would like to book a library pod. 'The pods are very nice and you can sit quietly and study very well . . . I come to the library to book space and there is no space for me to study . . . the main library is too big and I get easily distracted' (I, page 2, lines 13–15).

Although Participant I's struggles are less complex than those of Participant B, the individuals are finding studying difficult, leaving them at risk of not learning and engaging in the programme. Participant U stated: 'I would like more intervention – it makes a big difference in the understanding of the learning outcomes. I struggle with the basics of referencing and general essay writing; it really does hinder my learning and whether I pass my assessments or not. I have recently failed an assignment – I just didn't understand what I needed to do to pass' (U, page 2, lines 20–25).

Participant D, a learner from one of the satellite sites, is explicit in her interview: 'We need support with the basics of literacy and numeracy. The nursing course is not easy; I have recently sat my Maths Medicine exam and there were far too many words on the exam paper. I was distracted by the scenario; I didn't pass my exam and I now need more help please' (D, page 2, lines 49–53).

The interviews from a researcher's point of view were at times difficult to understand, and the level of resilience shown by these learners was incredible. Participant H is on her second attempt at her Medicine Management assessment, and the participant is scared of further failure: 'I am preparing for my exam. Maths for Nurses has been helpful, and I am learning, but still struggling to make sense of some of the math equations' (H, page 2, lines 15–18).

In summary, the subordinate theme 'Learner struggles' has shown that participants have difficult home lives where daily struggles and learning cause high levels of anxiety. Some participants explain that childcare, domestic violence, attending the family court, and financial difficulties can make learning impossible. The risk of attrition is high for these learners, and their individual struggles have meant not passing exams and having referrals in all types of assessment. Other divergences and convergences are space, time, lack of understanding, and the need for face-to-face learning.

LEARNER SUPPORT

This subordinate theme links to additional support for the learner undertaking undergraduate nursing. Each participant was able to express their support needs in their interviews. Six participants were able to discuss the additional support to help them to be successful learners.

Participant P stated, 'Ongoing support is needed for my assessments; without the support I will fail my module' (P, page 2, line 12). 'Intervention programmes are important and help us to plant our seeds for learning; we need to revise for our exams all the way. Some of us know we need to come for additional support' (P, page 2, lines 15–17).

Participant F backs up what Participant P is saying: 'Help and intervention makes a lot of difference to us as students; we want to learn and succeed. I want to overcome my language barrier' (F, page 2, lines 42–43).

Participant M had a clear insight for those learners she deemed to be underconfident in the classroom: 'People that don't speak up will attend extra classes and it will really help to build their confidence' (M, page 2, line 24).

Participant L has already started to attend some extra classes in Maths for Nurses. 'The Maths for Nurses group is positive, and I have learnt my drug calculations; I feel more confident' (L, page 2, line 39).

Interestingly, Participant E wants more intervention and can see the marketing but doesn't feel that the online and face-to-face interventions are equal to all students on the satellite sites: 'I know there is a Maths flyer on the main campus to improve literacy and numeracy, but it is face to face; this is a problem with the satellite campus . . . we don't feel as involved . . . I think sometimes we don't receive all the emails from our lecturers' (E, page 2, lines 37–41).

Participant G said: 'For me personally, extra support in maths is absolutely important so that I can finish my course; without the additional support I will fail' (G, page 2, line 17).

Participant C said in his interview, 'I would like help with interviewing skills so that I am able to be successful in finding a job' (C, page 2, line 44).

Participants are clear about the use of additional support to enhance their studies, and there is a 'knowing' amongst the learners about the importance of addressing underlying learning needs that may in the long term impede their overall learning success in their undergraduate nursing programme. By addressing their additional learning need the learners are effectively mitigating the risks of attrition.

In summary, in the subordinate theme 'Additional support', learners have demonstrated a clear sense of self and awareness and know that they can build their own agency with additional support. All participants were able to show how they were able to navigate additional support for themselves or were aware of where to source the support. Some learners were able to see a lack of parity where additional support classes were available. The learners in this sample had the self-awareness to address their learning needs and to seek support where required. Self-efficacy for these learners is evident from their individual interviews.

SUCCESS IN LEARNING

This subordinate theme links to the learning success experienced by undergraduate nurses. Some participants were able to discuss their lived experiences of what successful learning looked like to them as individual learners. Four participants were explicit in explaining how they found success and were able to describe the vehicles helping to drive their own successes.

Participant Q explained that they had a disability that at times hindered their learning outcomes. 'Success to me is passing my exams and becoming a registered nurse; I have always wanted to be a nurse and I won't let my disability get in my way. I have found the intervention group for Maths brilliant, and I have recently passed my Medicine Management on the second attempt. I feel so happy and successful' (Q, page 2, lines 28–35).

Participant O had recently been to the Maths for Nurses class and explained, 'I struggle with childcare so the lunchtime extra support for Maths has really worked for me. Passing my Maths exam in nursing for the second time has made me more confident for the future. I will be moving into year 3 of my nursing soon and I am hopeful that I will complete my course' (O, page 2, lines 18–25).

Participant S explained in the interview, 'Leap Online is really good – I zap the QR code and that's me booked into my extra Maths class. Understanding how the drugs calculations work has had a positive impact on my learning' (S, page 2, lines 21–29).

Participant K was clear about her learning and how she was going to achieve her learning outcomes. 'I like interventions like Maths and English; it breaks my learning into small steps. I am much better at doing my drug calculations now; strong support has given me a new learning target, and this make me feel confident. To finish my nursing degree is my main aim, and success in my assessments builds my confidence and gives me a boost for my career as a nurse. I am feeling more confident because of the help that I have received; I feel proud of myself' (K, page 2, lines 24–32).

In summary, the subordinate theme 'Success in learning' shows the participants in all cases to have said that they have benefitted from intervention to enhance their individual learning opportunities. At times their individual testimonies give rise to how happy they feel with small-step success in their learning and how much lighter they feel once their assessment on the second attempt has been achieved. The participants were able to understand how their confidence and self-efficacy have increased; these elements left the participants in this sample feeling more agentic and able to move forward with their future learning goals. Although learners had not discussed their own levels of resilience, the comments made by the participants have demonstrated high levels of resilience and sustainability, enabling new learning to take place.

Superordinate Theme (4): Successful Learning

The fourth superordinate theme, 'Successful learning', gives testimonies of how learners have engaged in the Maths for Nurses pilot programme. Learners were able to report on their maths starting points after their baseline maths assessment.

Under this theme, learners were able to discuss their learning journey of improvement, differentiation, and success after building new knowledge and understanding of maths used by the nursing professional for competence of medicine management and patient safety. This superordinate theme centres on four subordinate themes: (1) Learner starting point, (2) Learning journey, (3) Differentiation, and (4) Knowledge and understanding.

LEARNER STARTING POINT

This subordinate theme is centred on comments made by the undergraduate nurse learner at specific moments in their learning. Starting points are different for everyone. Seven participants discussed their starting points.

Participant Q said, 'Using my learning contract as a starting point has given a focus for myself, my lecturer, and also my personal tutor' (Q, page 3, lines 23–24).

Participant L explained to the researcher that she visualised her success in learning at the beginning of the course. 'I started my course by trying to believe in myself and what it would be like to be qualified as a nurse and supporting people. I thought to myself: if I don't pass I need to keep on trying until I do' (L, page 3, lines 43–46).

Participant P wanted to be successful for her family and explained how her starting points were important for each assessment and every new placement. 'Success to me means starting all my assessments and new [placements] with a strong and positive attitude towards my learning. I really want my family to be proud of me, so I start by always trying hard' (P, page 3, lines 21–23).

Participant A said, 'My starting points are to read everything very carefully. I like to have my module information with me at all times, so I don't forget what I am doing and also what is coming up that I need to action' (A, page 3, lines 26–28).

Participant I's interview comments were like those of Participants L and P: 'I think hard work always pays off. It is important that I start my studies by thinking that I want to be a good nurse; doing my best really matters to me and I want to make everyone around me feel proud of my efforts with my nursing degree' (I, page 3, lines 22–26).

Participants T and B were both saying the same, that they would like to start their module with lots of information to aid their overall success; the starting points were essential for successful learning outcomes.

In summary, 'Learner starting point' was deemed as being essential by each of the participants in the sample. For each participant, setting the scene for learning and being clear on their expected learning outcomes were both important aspects for successful learning, in both the short and long terms. Participants were able to see their end point, and all wanted to become qualified nurses and to make their families and lecturers proud of their individual efforts.

LEARNING JOURNEY

This subordinate theme, 'Learning journey', gives participants' comments on their learning journey so far and includes academic assessment and placement experiences. There were seven participants in this sample, and each had interesting and different stories of their learning journey.

Participant O states, 'I am on the child nursing course, and I have enjoyed my learning so far. I did have a difficult placement though, where I didn't feel that I received enough support; other nurses were too busy and short staffed, so I didn't think I had enough learning opportunities. At one point I did feel like leaving the course' (O, page 3, lines 31–33).

Participant S describes her learning journey as a positive one. 'I have received good assessment results and I am pleased with my learning outcomes; this hasn't always been the case until recently when I have accessed Maths for Nurses and academic writing support. I did pass my Anatomy and Physiology exam with a high mark and I am pleased with myself; my learning is going well and I think that I will complete the course. Six months ago, I wanted to pack it all in due to failed assessments and a difficult placement' (S, page 3, lines 34–37). Lack of support and learner dissatisfaction often play a part in the attrition of undergraduate nurses.

Participant G gives a different slant to their lived experiences whilst doing their undergraduate nursing studies. 'I did my Maths and English in Portugal – I didn't extend my learning straight away as I had a baby; my baby is older now . . . Doing my nursing course has been a positive journey – I am so grateful and I know that if I study hard I will be able to provide for my son as I am a single parent and money is tight' (G, page 3, lines 26–28).

Another interesting contrast in the participants' learning journeys is Participant J's ideas about learner success. 'You have to work smart as sometimes we are under a lot of pressure. I manage my time when my children are in bed; I go straight away and do some work. I wake up early when I don't have a class or just stay back at Uni if I can. If I want to be successful, I need to work hard' (J, page 3, lines 87–93). Participant J demonstrates high levels of motivation and resilience and has the knowledge and understanding of how to utilise time to aid learner success.

Participant R fully understood the importance of learner success. 'Success means a lot to me as I am progressing through the university and hopefully making good progress. I am passing my modules and enjoying my placements which have to date been successful. I am looking forward to the future using my university knowledge' (R, page 3, lines 30–32).

Participant U identified learner success as have a good learning time: 'I would say engaging in class and doing the best you can, whilst passing your essays and presentations and always trying your best' (U, page 3, lines 37–39).

Participant H finally summed up successful learning within her own learning narrative: 'When you are successful in your learning, you are going out from the university as a professional, having a good job in the competitive market' (H, page 3, lines 26–27).

In summary, 'Learning journey' was experienced differently by each participant. Participants in the sample discussed the positives and negatives of their own individual learning journey. Some described their disappointment with support on placements, whilst others were championing their successes. All participants in the sample could explain that an undergraduate nursing course can be tough and that application, concentration, and trying their best were the essence of successful learning, and enable the building of knowledge and understanding, leading to successful outcomes and completion of the nursing course. There was also an element of the learner experience where dissatisfaction can lead to attrition in the long term.

DIFFERENTIATION

The subordinate theme 'Differentiation' gives rise to additional support, one-to-one learning, and the differentiation of learner needs. There were four participants in the sample.

Participant N was able to say: 'One-to-one support is needed to progress my learning; I have no belief in the university service to give me the support I need. I have enquired and not heard anything back, so I don't know where to go next . . . a whole month has passed without support – I have attended the new Maths for Nurses group and this has helped me. I am going to attend the academic writing group next week' (N, page 3, lines 31–34). This participant was signposted to support on the same day of the interview; the learner was frustrated and needed more one-to-one support.

Participant K explained, 'Intervention support has improved my self-esteem and I feel self-accomplishment; my language has developed, and my written English skills have improved' (K, page 3, lines 48–50).

Participant E discussed her struggles and felt that a good performance coupled with encouraging feedback from her teacher would help her learning journey: 'If I struggle and don't get 100% in [the] Medicine Management module, I will need good feedback and ongoing support or I will definitely fail again' (E, page 3, lines 56–58).

Participant D gave clear reasons in her interview why differentiation and support are important in her individual case: 'I am already a qualified nurse in Greece, so I know what it feels like to be successful; however, I have many health issues, personal issues, and problems with finance – this can all affect my learning processes. I have failed some of my first modules due to my mum having a stroke; I have become her carer' (D, page 3, lines 85–89).

In summary, 'Differentiation' is essential for some learners, and without the differentiation of learning, the learner will struggle and become dissatisfied, leading to attrition. The learners in the sample could all explain the importance of individual support to aid successful learning outcomes.

In one case the participant was supported immediately to ensure that one-to-one support was available; the learner went on to achieve successful learning outcomes. Assessment of learning needs and learner contracts are essential in ensuring that the learner is supported in their undergraduate nursing studies.

KNOWLEDGE AND UNDERSTANDING

In the subordinate theme 'Knowledge and understanding', the participants were able to state how knowledge is built and why understanding is important for successful learning. There were three participants in this sample.

Participant C said that building knowledge and understanding 'is about having the confidence to ask questions to deepen thinking and learning; also taking advantage of everything that is given to us as students to enhance our learning' (C, page 3, line 49).

Participant M gave similar information: 'Successful learning is building knowledge and understanding of the topic, understanding the course and being confident using new skills in practice' (M, page 3, lines 28–29).

Participant F again reiterated what was said by Participants C and M: 'Successful learning is when it has changed our attitude, when it has also changed our behaviour towards learning. Gaining proper skills, this is learning success and not superficial' (F, page 3, lines 47–48).

In summary, knowledge and understanding was understood by a small sample of learners. The participants in this sample were able to say that when knowledge and understanding is scaffold, the learning will take place. The new learning builds confidence and self-esteem, leading to change in learning behaviour and attitude. The evidence from the participants further demonstrates an increase in motivation and self-efficacy.

Superordinate Theme (5): Sense of Self

The fifth superordinate theme, 'Sense of self', demonstrated participants explaining their individual learning growth and moments of epiphany. Under this theme, learners were explicit when explaining their increased sense of self and how some participants have become more agentic when embarking on the Maths for Nurses pilot programme. This superordinate theme gives four important subordinate themes: (1) Learner growth, (2) Moments of epiphany, (3) Increased sense of self, and (4) Becoming more agentic.

LEARNER GROWTH

In this subordinate theme, the participants were able to explain their own individual learning growth. Six of the participants in the sample were able to describe their learning growth and how the scaffold learning made them feel.

Participant D said, 'Interventions for students are helpful; I would like to see more support as my learning and confidence have really grown. My grades have improved, and I am on the right track with additional support from my personal tutor' (D, page 3, lines 122–124).

Participant J had a lot to say about learning growth for her as an individual: 'My course is building my confidence and if you are confident, you understand maths because maths is not something you grasp straight away. You have to practise your skills like you do with everything in life; if I understand the teacher then I make less mistakes. I am feeling more confident than I did at the beginning of the course' (J, page 2, lines 102–105).

Participant U emulated the learning growth of Participants D and J: 'I am attending an English class to improve my referencing—I will feel more confident if it goes well. I have seen intervention build the confidence of my friend who has many children and was struggling before she had the help' (U, page 3, lines 52–54).

Participant I showed levels of motivation when new learning had taken place: 'Being part of an intervention group has helped me to interact with other students. I know I am not the only one feeling nervous about my maths; I don't feel isolated. Having intervention sessions face to face has really helped and is much better than online, and you can have one-to-one additional learning too. When I interact face to face, I learn new things; communication has been key to my growth in my learning' (I, page 3, lines 32–36).

Participant A also reiterated, 'One-to-one learning is good in Maths for Nurses – I have learnt so much, and I can now do my calculations whereas I couldn't before the classes' (A, page 3, line 60).

Participant K further reinforced learner growth by stating, 'I have really grown in the past two years, and I am proud of myself . . . It has not been easy juggling children and all the travel' (K, page 3, lines 59–60).

In summary, 'Learner growth' has been a positive experience for several undergraduate nurses. The sample participants could comment on the intervention programmes available for undergraduate nurses to develop their literacy and numeracy skills. The role of the personal tutor is supportive and key to learner growth. Participants were able to talk about being less nervous regarding their maths anxiety and did not feel so isolated. Some participants preferred face-to-face learning for their intervention work and had become more confident and prouder that they had passed their assessments.

MOMENTS OF EPIPHANY

In this subordinate theme, participants discussed their 'lightbulb moments' and times of enlightenment or surprise. There were seven participants in this sample, who spoke eloquently about their special moments in their learning journey.

Participant O said, 'I think by the time I have completed my Maths for Nurses sessions . . . I can see what I am struggling with for moving forward; opening an exam paper can be overwhelming, but you can see that everyone is in the same boat. It has been the light at the end of tunnel . . . it was good progress in the end' (O, page 3, lines 34–38).

Participant N was able to see that she needed more support. 'I have found learning primitive and basic in clinical skills and academic work too hard; I need to build my confidence further in my academic learning' (N, page 3, lines 62–64).

Participant E explained that she would like more monitoring of her learning: 'We need frequent check-ups, to see how we are doing and reassurance that we are doing great. The first year of my undergraduate studies was on Zoom – this didn't feel personal enough – as soon as we were working face to face, I was much more confident' (E, page 3, lines 69–71).

Participant R was thoughtful and said, 'If I am not able to set my goals in the end, it will be a barrier to my learning; this will set me back because I want to achieve' (R, page 3, line 36).

Participant T reinforced the sentiments of the other participants in this sample by merely stating, 'Electronic working is not for me; I work better face to face and feel more confident. I have found new levels of confidence doing formulas and calculations face to face in the Maths for Nurses group' (T, page 3, lines 56–58).

Participant L was explicit when discussing small group work and having her learner voice heard. 'I have started to engage more easily in small groups; I think communication is a key skill that keeps us fully engaged and that is why I prefer small group learning. In big groups some people's voices are heard and it doesn't give a chance for other less confident people to speak. I don't always have a voice and my language barrier is hard in bigger groups; this is why the Maths for Nurses group has worked for me and I have recently passed my exam on the second attempt' (L, page 3, lines 53–63).

Finally, Participant C stated, 'I have seen students drop off the programme due to not understanding what is expected as a nurse. Some students have also fallen pregnant and not completed the course' (C, page 3, lines 65–66).

In summary, 'Moments of epiphany' has allowed participants to share important moments in their learning and how these moments have led to further learning and challenge, giving the participant a sense of self and the opportunity for new possibilities within their individual learning journey.

INCREASED SENSE OF SELF

In the subordinate theme 'Increased sense of self', participants in their interviews were able to explain to the researcher how their sense of self started to change during their undergraduate nursing programme. There were four participants in this sample.

Participant B explained, 'We are given a lot of reassurance – you know when you are on the right track . . . if you don't have some intervention, you may go off the track completely. Some of us are more mature, so intervention is good as we have mostly been out of learning for a while; we also have busy home lives. Our learning helps us to become who we want to be: professional people doing a good caring job' (B, page 3, lines 56–58).

Participant P was able to see an increased sense of self. 'The support I have been given since January is unbelievable; it has helped me a lot. It has also made me more confident and wanting to succeed so much' (P, page 3, lines 30–31).

In a similar vein, Participant M was able to discuss skill development within her nursing programme: 'One-to-one learning can support our skill development [to be] ready for our practice placement . . . it gives you a better sense of yourself and your capabilities when caring for other people in our communities' (M, page 3, lines 40–42).

Participant S said, 'Support and reassurance in learning and assessment and university and on placement 'have' increased my overall confidence' (S, page 3, lines 45–46).

In summary, an increased sense of self has been evident in the four participants' samples; support, reassurance, and intervention are the key themes discussed. One-to-one learning was further discussed, and the learners felt an increased sense of self during either group interventions or one-to-one support sessions. Successful learning and ongoing support to become a good caring nurse were also elements of the discussion and interpretation by the researchers.

BECOMING MORE AGENTIC

The subordinate theme 'Becoming more agentic' has been a time of change and development for participants. There were four participants in the sample, who felt that they had become more agentic.

Participant G discussed the fact that they could see people at the same level of themselves during the programme. 'It made me feel more confident that we could share the same common ground and also similar learning needs, so we could work together as a team to produce good learning outcomes' (G, page 3, lines 37–40).

Participant H said, 'When the university offers support, we are confident and we will do well; we become more authentic in our profession' (H, page 3, lines 30–32).

Participant Q further explained they had become more confident with their studies and felt that their learning contract had helped them to move forward with their studies. 'I have become more confident because I now have full support with my studies' (Q, page 3, line 61).

Participant F articulated, 'Nursing makes a huge difference to your confidence and self-esteem. I feel more confident now [that] I am in year 3 of my studies; I feel happy and proud of myself' (F, page 3, lines 55–57).

In summary, becoming more agentic during an undergraduate nursing course has been essential to the four participants in the sample. Everyone has demonstrated a true sense of self, and each participant has become more agentic, increasing their long-term agency for a successful career in the nursing profession. Self-efficacy has also increased for each learner in the sample.

Working collaboratively and teamworking are common themes within the sample.

Superordinate Theme (6): Learner at Risk Beliefs

The sixth superordinate theme, 'Learner at risk beliefs', gives statements from participants whereby they explain their existing beliefs regarding their individual learning processes and how they think the university staff perceive their learning and success. Within this theme, some learner participants could describe their learning outcomes that have been met or unmet and their individual perceptions.

This superordinate theme gives three subordinate themes: (1) Student-perceived beliefs, (2) Perceived beliefs about staff, and (3) Learning outcomes and met/unmet perceptions.

STUDENT-PERCEIVED BELIEFS

The subordinate theme 'Student-perceived beliefs' has been discussed with many variables and beliefs held by the participants. There were 10 participants in this sample, all holding strong beliefs regarding their undergraduate nursing studies, and some participants were able to identify any risk to their learning, and also where the participant could see positive learning, progress, and learning outcomes in assessment.

Participant T, who has a learning contract, was fully aware of her learning difficulties and stated, 'My belief is that I work much more productively when having my lectures and personal tutor sessions face to face; this is much better for my learning difficulties' (T, page 4, lines 86–87).

Participant P said that support is invaluable: 'A good level of support helps us to be successful in our learning; family issues and juggling childcare can hinder my learning at times, and in the past has been the reason that I have failed a module' (P, page 4, lines 73–74).

Participant E's interview was aligned with Participants T and P: 'We work better face to face and online learning hinders our engagement with each other so we can't check out with each other; I see this as a problem' (E, page 4, line 89).

Participant S was able to explain that 'intervention supports my learning and I believe that my language barrier can put me at risk of not always understanding my assessments' (S, page 4, line 79).

Participant D believed that she was at risk due to her financial situation. 'I would like to work and learn how to improve my finances. I worry about my money and children, and I am at risk of not completing my studies; this makes me very upset and sometimes I don't know what to do' (D, page 4, lines 82–83). The increase of travel and living costs is of interest to the researchers and will formulate into action planning and recommendations from the research.

Participant B stated in interview, 'I believe if you are mature you can cope with childcare and financial issues and you can attend intervention classes so that you don't get behind with your studies. English is my second language; I struggle with everything really, but I keep on going' (B, page 4, lines 76–78).

Participant A said that she was at risk from not learning because she finds it hard to find a quiet space to learn. 'I can't stay over at the Uni because I help my mum with her five children that are all younger than me; the house is so noisy; I believe this is why I failed my last assessment due to lack of preparation' (A, page 4, lines 65–66).

Participant L is hopeful in completing the undergraduate nursing course and believes this: 'Small groups make me more confident; I like how the nursing course is set up, but I would like more face-to-face teaching to extend the learning and to become more interactive' (L, page 4, lines 86–87).

Participant R, who is following the apprenticeship route in mental health nursing, believes this: 'Successful learning means a lot to me and much of my learning is online; I like this type of learning, but some other students I know feel isolated, and don't feel they learn as much virtually' (R, page 4, lines 36–37).

Finally, Participant O believed this: 'Engaging with the programme increases motivation and helps us to learn. I need additional help with my learning; if I didn't have the extra support I would fail my assessments' (O, page 4, line 89).

In summary, this subordinate theme, 'Student-perceived beliefs', has been illuminating and highlights how and why some learners may be at risk of attrition and not completing their 3-year undergraduate nursing course. Issues such as financial constraints and childcare struggles, family complications, language barriers, and online learning have been identified by the learners as hotspots that lead to difficulties in learning and that often affect learner attendance at university, online, and whilst on placement.

In contrast, other learners were able to identify successful learning through intervention programmes and have clearly stated that without the intervention, they would find their studies difficult due to language barriers and lack of assessment understanding.

PERCEIVED BELIEFS ABOUT STAFF

In this subordinate theme, "Perceived beliefs about staff", learners who were interviewed were able to discuss their beliefs about lecturers and placement staff in their undergraduate nursing course. There were seven participants in this sample.

Participant I said, 'Having a family makes you split two ways; I have a baby and I have to fit university into my time. University is supportive, but I want my assessment to be explained to me clearly; it is not always clear and this hinders my learning when I am juggling so many things' (I, page 4, lines 60–63).

Participant K explained, 'Personal tutors and Maths and English support help when English is not your first language. I find lecturers to be patient, but extra help is needed to understand assessment. I have met my recent learning outcomes with support' (K, page 4, lines 75–77).

Participant N, who has additional support and a learning contract in place, has thought about the length of the undergraduate nursing course: 'I think the course is too long; we are not stretched enough in the area of clinical skills and I believe academic work is difficult; I prefer the practical side' (N, page 4, lines 78–79).

Participant Q said, 'I struggle with learning and believe that I need more help; I find it hard to speak up' (Q, page 4, line 56).

Participant H emulated Participant N and stated, 'With more help and support, we become more confident; I believe if we don't have enough support then it does have consequences. I have seen people leave the programme; we want tutors to understand our needs as students' (H, page 4, lines 81–82).

Participant F said, 'I want to see more support for bilingual learners and better access to all information about learning on one page' (F, page 4, lines 59–60).

Finally, Participant G explained this in the interview: 'Written assessments are a barrier to learning if not discussed clearly; learning steps need to be broken down to aid understanding. I have enjoyed my most recent intervention class, "Maths for Nurses"' (G, page 4, lines 69–70).

In summary, 'Perceived beliefs about staff' has produced findings relating to planning, preparation, and assessment rubrics. Some participants would prefer small-step learning and more practical-based assessment to support learning and language barriers. There is some evidence in this subordinate theme suggesting that lack of support can lead to undergraduate nursing learner attrition.

LEARNING OUTCOMES AND MET/UNMET PERCEPTIONS

In the subordinate theme 'Learning outcomes and met/unmet perceptions', learners were able to express their own views of their met or unmet learning needs. There were three participants in this sample.

Participant J explained, 'Being dyslexic does affect my learning and writing and I know that if I listen to lectures carefully, I will learn more, but my writing is still an issue. If you don't understand the course or assessments, it does affect your motivation to continue. I think assessment can be confusing if not explained and has in the past led to me failing an assessment' (J, page 4, lines 78–79).

Participant M said, 'One-to-one support helps me understand clinical skill development. I have experienced a good intervention group; I have been successful in my last maths exam' (M, page 4, line 76).

Participant C explained, 'I learn a lot from being hands on and also by observing other nurses in practice; this has helped me to pass my placements successfully' (C, page 4, line 73).

In summary, 'Learning outcomes and met/unmet perceptions' has been analysed and discussed by a small sample of learners from the whole sample. The small sample indicated individual pearls of success and demonstrates how individual undergraduate nurses can understand their own levels of learning to enable the learner to scaffold their own learning for future success at the end of the 3-year programme.

Superordinate Theme (7): Relationship Beliefs and Practice

The seventh superordinate theme, 'Relationship beliefs and practice', relates to the participants' experience of feedforward feedback and the participants' journey of moving forward. Within this theme, learner participants are able to cite the strengths and weaknesses in their individual relationship beliefs and how this links to the practice that learners have experienced for themselves during the undergraduate nursing programme as a learner. This superordinate theme has three subordinate themes: (1) Feedforward feedback, (2) Strengths and weaknesses, and (3) Learner success.

FEEDFORWARD FEEDBACK

The subordinate theme 'Feedforward feedback' reviews the learners' views of feedback in support of their learning outcomes. The participants in the sample were making similar statements and were able to see the importance of good relationship building via quality feedback between the lecturer and the learners studying undergraduate nursing. There were nine participants in the sample, and each individual had a different angle on their view of feedback.

Participant L stated, 'More face-to-face learning will build relationships further and good clear feedback helps me learn better, so that I don't make the same mistakes twice' (L, page 4, line 87).

Participant A held a similar view of feedback and said that 'without feedback I would most definitely fail some of my assessment; I really value formative feedback' (A, page 4, line 78).

Participant B discussed the importance of self-confidence: 'Good formative feedback is essential and is a good confidence builder for assessment success. Any additional input from personal tutors and module teachers does make a difference in the teacher–student relationship and success in learning' (B, page 4, line 89).

Building good relationships resonated with Participant J: 'Good relationships with lecturers make a big difference; we want lecturers to listen carefully to our language needs to enable us to receive good quality feedback' (J, page 4, line 77).

Participant M wanted to address her strengths and weaknesses: 'Feedback is essential and helps us to address our weaknesses and develop our strengths' (M, page 4, line 67).

Participant C had a good insight into transferable skills: 'I have used my transferable skills to build teamwork and good relations with my fellow students' (C, page 4, line 67). The interview evidence has demonstrated how relationship building and good-quality feedback resonate with each other to produce an increase in communication, good teaching and learning, and informative assessment.

Participant N, with additional needs, said, 'More feedback is needed – more help in the first year of our studies is essential if you have a language barrier and a learning disability' (N, page 4, line 88).

Participant K had similar difficulties with their learning. 'I always ask for feedback to help with my learning; some of my friends don't and I know this affects their learning' (K, page 4, line 91).

Finally, Participant H said, 'I would like to be listened to by my tutors; I need more help and feedback' (H, page 4, line 59).

In summary, this subordinate theme, 'Feedforward feedback', has provided the researchers with a rich collage of participant comment and therefore gives the researchers a good knowledge and understanding of why relationship building between the lecturer and learner is essential even before any feedforward feedback is given to the undergraduate nurse during their programme of study.

Another theme clearly coming through as a golden thread is the idea that excellent feedforward feedback is a confidence builder, and the assessment infrastructure can help to build learner success during the 3-year course.

STRENGTHS AND WEAKNESSES

The subordinate theme 'Strengths and weaknesses' has some similar learner comments and other comments that are unique to this particular theme. There were seven participants in this sample.

Participant G said this about their own strengths and weaknesses: 'I understand my own language difficulties and I want lots of help with my assessments. I have attended the Maths for Nurses intervention group to improve my understanding of medicine management and patient safety. I strive to be successful and want to complete my studies' (G, page 4, lines 66–67.)

Participant E discussed good relationship building: 'I am able to confide in my personal tutor and we have a good relationship. I think face-to-face learning and [having a] contract have created better relationships for us all' (E, page 4, line 82).

Participant F talked about respect: 'I think I have a good relationship with my tutors; I am always respectful to them, and I always find the right support. I just ask, and they are always on my side' (F, page 4, line 67).

Participants P, T, D, and S stated that support was crucial to their learning and that it is the ongoing support from personal tutors that helps them to become successful learners.

In summary, the theme 'Strengths and weaknesses' gives the researchers an indication of the mixed ingredients of support required by the undergraduate nurse learner when it comes to addressing their own individual strengths and weaknesses. The sample of participant interviews gives an idea of how the learners are resilient and creative in developing strategies to address their own learning needs.

LEARNER SUCCESS

In the subordinate theme 'Learner success', the sample is small; nevertheless, participants were able to express the most important elements of successful learning.

Participant O said, 'I think the lecturer and student relationship needs to grow to facilitate good teaching, learning and assessment' (O, page 4, line 81).

Participant R's testimony was similar: 'Having a good relationship with my personal tutor and module teachers is essential to my overall learning' (R, page 4, line 59).

Participant U enjoyed the support they received from their personal tutor. 'Personal tutor support has been brilliant and has helped to foster a good relationship between my academic progress and the signposting I have received for my personal issues that have now resolved thanks to the support I have received' (U, page 4, line 62).

Participant I said, 'When I lost my ID badge, I was worried; staff were supportive and replaced my badge. The care at the university is good and the little things have made a real difference to me personally such as cheap meals and drink when I have very little money' (I, page 4, line 91).

Participant Q, who has a disability, stated, 'I have a disability that is hidden; my success has been due to the Leap Online sessions that I have attended' (Q, page 4, line 67).

In summary, the subordinate theme 'Learner success' has come in many guises, and although the sample is small, it is easy for the researchers to understand that the university is supportive of learning and the services for the learners are working in terms of additional support carried forward with a caring attitude that is learner focused.

CHAPTER 6

The Consequences of Attrition on Undergraduate Nurses: A Critical Analysis

Amanda Costello

Introduction

Attrition among undergraduate nursing students is a pressing issue that has far-reaching implications for the healthcare sector. It refers to the premature withdrawal of students from their nursing programmes before completion, which affects not only the students but also educational institutions, healthcare systems, and patient care outcomes. High attrition rates can lead to a shortage of qualified nurses, increased financial burdens, and emotional distress among students and faculty members. This chapter critically examines the consequences of attrition among undergraduate nurses, considering its impact on students, educational institutions, healthcare facilities, and the wider society.

Impact on Students

Attrition has profound personal and professional implications for students who leave their nursing programmes prematurely.

EMOTIONAL AND PSYCHOLOGICAL IMPACT

- Many students experience feelings of failure, disappointment, and lowered self-esteem.
- Leaving a programme can lead to anxiety and depression, especially if students struggle to find alternative career paths.
- The social stigma associated with dropping out may affect their confidence in pursuing further education or employment.

Leaving a university programme can have deep emotional and psychological consequences. Many students report feelings of failure, lowered self-esteem, and significant distress upon discontinuation. These effects are compounded by the challenge of finding new career paths and by the social stigma that often surrounds dropping out.

Furthermore, students who leave their programmes often internalise their experience as personal failure. In a UK-wide survey reported by *The Independent*, 'Half of students who dropped out said they felt like a failure, and the same proportion regretted their decision to leave university' (Griffiths, 2020, p. 6). This internalised failure can reduce a student's self-worth and belief in their academic and professional potential.

Additionally, the stigma of not completing higher education continues to carry significant weight. In one study, '44% of students reported a lack of confidence after dropping out, and 58% experienced depression,' (Griffiths, 2020, p. 7) illustrating the potent emotional consequences of academic withdrawal.

Mental health issues are both a cause and a consequence of dropping out. According to a study published in *The Lancet Public Health*, 'young people who are in higher education in England face a small increased risk of depression and anxiety, compared to their peers who are not attending higher education' (UCL, 2023, p. 2). The psychological strain of university, coupled with the stress of leaving, can lead to enduring anxiety and depressive episodes.

These findings are supported by a Gallup-Lumina study, which stated: 'Three in five undergraduates cited emotional stress and mental health as a reason for stopping coursework' (Gallup & Lumina Foundation, 2023, p. 8). The transition from university life can leave students without the support networks on which they previously relied, deepening their emotional isolation.

Social perceptions about educational success create a stigma around dropping out, which can further impact a student's confidence and willingness to reengage in education or employment. As Verywell Health (2023, p. 12) reports, 'stigma contributes to feelings of shame, social withdrawal, and reduced opportunities for recovery and reintegration.' This social burden may discourage former students from returning to academia or pursuing competitive job markets due to fear of judgement or perceived inadequacy.

These effects can persist long after the initial decision to leave has been made, affecting not only mental health but also long-term socioeconomic outcomes.

The decision to leave university is rarely made lightly, and the emotional and psychological impacts are often profound and multifaceted. Feelings of failure, anxiety, depression, and social stigma are common and underscore the importance of robust institutional support systems. Universities must prioritise accessible mental health resources and actively work to destigmatise alternative educational pathways, helping students to find renewed purpose beyond traditional academic success.

FINANCIAL CONSEQUENCES

- Tuition fees, student loans, and other financial investments may go to waste when a student drops out.
- Students may face difficulty repaying loans without the anticipated income from a nursing career.

Additional expenses may arise if students decide to reenrol in another programme. Leaving a university programme, particularly in fields like nursing, entails significant financial repercussions that can affect students' economic stability and future prospects. These consequences include the potential loss of tuition fees and student loans, challenges in loan repayment without the anticipated income from a nursing career, and additional expenses if reenrolling in another academic programme.

When a student withdraws from their course, they may still be liable for tuition fees corresponding to the period attended. In the UK, tuition fees can be substantial, and students often finance them through loans. According to NHS Employers (2022), students begin repaying these loans once their income exceeds the repayment threshold, which is currently £27,295 per year. However, if a student leaves their programme prematurely, they may not achieve the qualification necessary to secure employment that meets this threshold, complicating repayment efforts.

The inability to complete a nursing degree can hinder access to registered nursing positions, which typically offer salaries above the repayment threshold. Without this anticipated income, repaying student loans becomes more challenging. Furthermore, any Maintenance Loan received is reassessed upon withdrawal. If the loan covers a period beyond the student's attendance, it is considered an overpayment and must be repaid immediately (GOV.UK, n.d.). This immediate financial obligation can place additional strain on students who may already be facing economic hardship.

Students who decide to reenrol in another academic programme may encounter further financial burdens. Eligibility for student finance can be affected by previous study, potentially limiting access to loans or grants for the new course. The University of Bradford (n.d.) notes that students must pay a minimum of 50% of their fees to complete reenrolment unless covered by a sponsor or student finance. This upfront cost can be a significant barrier for those seeking to continue their education.

The financial implications of leaving a nursing programme are multifaceted and substantial. They encompass the potential loss of invested tuition fees and loans, difficulties in loan repayment without the expected income, and additional costs associated with reenrolment. Prospective students should carefully consider these factors and seek comprehensive financial advice before making decisions about withdrawing from their studies.

CAREER DISRUPTIONS

- Those who drop out may struggle to find well-paying jobs due to their incomplete qualifications.
- They may need to transition into lower-paying or unrelated fields, limiting career advancement opportunities.
- Some students may reattempt nursing education, but the loss of time and motivation can hinder their progress.

Leaving a nursing programme before completion can lead to significant career disruptions, affecting employment opportunities, earning potential, and professional development. These challenges include difficulties in securing well-paying jobs due to incomplete qualifications, the necessity to transition into lower-paying or unrelated fields, and obstacles faced when reattempting nursing education.

Individuals who leave nursing programmes without obtaining a degree often encounter barriers when seeking employment in the healthcare sector. The absence of formal qualifications limits access to registered nursing positions which typically offer higher salaries and career stability. Consequently, these individuals may find themselves in roles that do not utilise their partial training, leading to underemployment and financial strain. As noted by the American Association of Colleges of Nursing (AACN), a decline in nursing programme enrolments raises concerns about the nursing workforce, indicating that incomplete education exacerbates existing skill shortages and employment challenges in the field (AACN, 2023).

Without the credentials conferred by a nursing degree, former students may need to explore employment opportunities outside of healthcare. This transition often involves accepting positions with lower remuneration and limited prospects for advancement. The Urban Institute highlights that educational attainment significantly influences career trajectories, with incomplete education restricting access to higher-paying roles and professional growth (Spetz & Bates, 2013). Such shifts can lead to decreased job satisfaction and financial instability, impacting on long-term career goals. Therefore, some individuals may choose to reenrol in nursing programmes to complete their education. However, this path presents its own set of challenges. The time away from formal education can result in a loss of academic momentum and confidence, making the return to rigorous study demanding. Research indicates that students who take breaks from their studies often face difficulties in reengagement, with factors such as diminished motivation and external obligations hindering their progress (Wang & Baker, 2018). Additionally, policies regarding readmission vary among institutions, and previous academic performance may influence the likelihood of acceptance. Financial constraints also play a role, as returning students may have exhausted available funding or incurred debts from prior enrolment periods.

The decision to leave a nursing programme before completion carries substantial career implications, including limited employment opportunities, potential shifts to less desirable job sectors, and challenges associated with reentering educational pathways. Prospective students should carefully consider these factors and seek academic and career counselling to make informed decisions about their educational pursuits.

Impact on Educational Institutions

Attrition rates also affect nursing schools and universities, often negatively influencing academic programmes and institutional reputations.

FINANCIAL LOSSES

- Institutions lose tuition revenue when students drop out, which can affect funding for faculty salaries, infrastructure, and academic resources.

Government funding and accreditation bodies often assess universities based on student retention rates, meaning that student attrition in higher education institutions has significant financial ramifications, affecting tuition revenue, resource allocation, and funding from governmental and accreditation bodies.

When students withdraw from their studies prematurely, universities experience a direct loss in tuition income. In the UK, with average tuition fees around £9000 per year, a dropout rate of 6.3% equates to an annual financial loss of approximately £1.62 billion across institutions (FE News Editor, 2023). This reduction in revenue can constrain budgets allocated for faculty salaries, infrastructure development, and the enhancement of academic resources. As noted by Coates and Petts (2024), universities are heavily dependent on tuition fees, which account for more than half of their funding. Consequently, any decline in student numbers directly impacts the financial stability of these institutions.

Governmental funding bodies often assess universities based on student retention and completion rates. In England, the Office for Students (OfS) employs a funding model where allocations are influenced by student numbers and retention metrics. Institutions failing to meet agreed-upon student completion targets may face financial penalties or reduced funding (House of Commons Public Accounts Committee, 2008). Furthermore, high attrition rates can adversely affect a university's performance metrics in frameworks such as the Teaching Excellence and Student Outcomes Framework (TEF), potentially influencing accreditation status and future funding opportunities (Teaching Excellence Framework, n.d.).

Beyond the immediate loss of tuition fees, student attrition contributes to broader financial challenges within the higher education sector. Bolton and Lewis (2025) report that nearly three-quarters (72%) of higher education providers could be in deficit by 2025–2026, with declining student numbers being a significant contributing factor. This financial strain may necessitate cost-cutting measures, including staff redundancies and programme closures, further impacting the quality of education and institutional reputation.

High student dropout rates pose substantial financial challenges for universities, leading to decreased tuition revenue and potential reductions in government funding. These financial strains can adversely affect faculty compensation, infrastructure projects, and the availability of academic resources. Addressing student retention is therefore crucial for the financial sustainability and overall quality of higher education institutions.

REPUTATION AND ACCREDITATION

- High attrition rates can damage the credibility of nursing programmes, making it harder to attract new students.
- Poor retention rates impact an institution's ability to offer nursing degrees.

Accreditation bodies may impose stricter regulations on institutions with high attrition rates in nursing programmes. This can significantly undermine their credibility, making it challenging to attract prospective students and potentially leading to stricter regulations from accreditation bodies.

High dropout rates within nursing programmes can tarnish their reputation, deterring potential applicants. A study by Merkley (2016) highlighted that attrition rates in some baccalaureate nursing programmes can reach as high as 50%, raising concerns about programme effectiveness and stability. Such statistics may lead prospective students to question the quality and support offered by these programmes, thereby reducing enrolment numbers. Furthermore, the AACN (2023) reported a 1.4% decrease in entry-level baccalaureate nursing programme enrolments, ending a 20-year growth trend, suggesting that perceptions of programme instability may influence the application rate.

Accreditation organisations closely monitor student retention and graduation rates as indicators of programme quality. The National Council of State Boards of Nursing (NCSBN) emphasises that performance outcomes, including graduation rates, are critical metrics used by boards of nursing and other accrediting entities (Spector et al., 2018). Programmes exhibiting poor retention may face intensified scrutiny and be required to implement corrective measures to maintain accreditation status. Accreditation standards often drive curriculum and educational changes, with accreditors expecting programmes to meet established benchmarks to ensure quality education (Halstead, 2022). Failure to comply with these standards can result in limitations on the institution's ability to offer nursing degrees, thereby affecting its academic standing and financial health.

High attrition rates in nursing programmes not only damage their credibility and hinder student recruitment but also invite stricter oversight from accreditation bodies. Maintaining low attrition is essential for preserving programme reputation, attracting qualified applicants, and ensuring compliance with accrediting standards.

STRAIN ON FACULTY AND RESOURCES

- Faculty members may experience burnout when they invest time and effort in students who eventually drop out.
- Resources allocated to struggling students may not yield long-term benefits if attrition rates remain high.
- A large percentage of students fail to complete their studies.

The overall effectiveness of the nursing curriculum may be questioned if high attrition rates in nursing programmes significantly impact faculty well-being, resource allocation, and perceptions of curriculum effectiveness.

Faculty members invest considerable time and effort in educating nursing students. When students drop out, this investment may seem futile, leading to emotional exhaustion and burnout. A study by Zangaro et al. (2023) found that 85.2% of nursing faculty reported moderate to high levels of burnout, highlighting the widespread nature of this issue. Factors contributing to burnout include high workloads, unsupported environments, and job dissatisfaction (Ulmen & Lloyd, 2023).

Resources allocated to support struggling students may not yield long-term benefits if attrition rates remain high. High attrition rates decrease the number of nursing school graduates, contributing to the shortage of nursing professionals

(Kukkonen et al., 2023). This inefficiency not only affects the institution's financial stability but also hampers efforts to address the broader nursing shortage.

Persistent high attrition rates may lead to scrutiny of the nursing curriculum's effectiveness. Attrition rates among nursing students are a global issue and a possible factor in current nursing shortages (Georgieva et al., 2024). Such perceptions can damage the programme's reputation, making it less attractive to prospective students and stakeholders.

High student attrition in nursing programmes places significant strain on faculty, leads to inefficient use of resources, and raises concerns about curriculum effectiveness. Addressing these challenges is crucial for improving faculty well-being, optimising resource utilisation, and enhancing the quality and reputation of nursing education.

The healthcare sector heavily relies on nursing graduates to fill workforce gaps. Attrition among undergraduate nurses significantly disrupts this balance.

NURSING SHORTAGES

- High attrition rates contribute to an inadequate supply of qualified nurses, exacerbating workforce shortages in hospitals and clinics.
- Healthcare facilities may struggle to meet patient care demands, leading to increased workloads for existing staff.

High attrition rates in nursing education programmes significantly contribute to the ongoing shortage of qualified nurses, adversely affecting healthcare delivery and patient outcomes.

The departure of students from nursing programmes before completion directly diminishes the pool of new nurses entering the workforce. This exacerbates existing shortages, particularly as experienced nurses retire or leave the profession. The AACN reported a 1.4% decrease in enrolments for entry-level baccalaureate nursing programmes, ending a 20-year growth trend and raising concerns about the future supply of registered nurses (AACN, 2023). Such enrolment declines, coupled with high attrition rates, hinder efforts to address the growing demand for nursing professionals.

Nursing shortages compel healthcare facilities to operate with reduced staff, leading to increased workloads for existing nurses. This situation elevates stress levels and the risk of burnout among nursing staff. The Agency for Healthcare Research and Quality (AHRQ) has noted that inadequate nurse staffing is associated with missed nursing care and negative patient outcomes, including increased patient mortality (Boston-Leary et al., 2024). Furthermore, the NCSBN projected that by 2027, nearly 900,000 nurses intend to leave the workforce, potentially threatening the stability of the national healthcare system (NCSBN, 2023).

High attrition rates in nursing education programmes significantly contribute to the shortage of qualified nurses, adversely affecting healthcare facilities' ability to meet patient care demands and increasing workloads for existing staff. Addressing factors that lead to student attrition is crucial for ensuring a robust nursing workforce capable of delivering quality patient care.

INCREASED BURNOUT AMONG EXISTING STAFF

- Fewer nursing graduates means that current nurses must take on more responsibilities, leading to physical and mental exhaustion.
- Further worsening of the shortage crisis is predicted.

Burnout can result in higher turnover rates among working nurses. High attrition rates in nursing education programmes contribute to a reduced influx of new graduates into the healthcare system, leading to increased workloads for existing staff. This escalation in responsibilities can result in physical and mental exhaustion, commonly referred to as burnout. Burnout is characterised by emotional exhaustion, depersonalisation, and a diminished sense of personal accomplishment, adversely affecting both nurses and patient care quality.

The shortage of nursing graduates necessitates that current nurses assume additional duties, intensifying their workloads. This heightened demand can lead to significant physical and mental fatigue. Internationally, a study published in the *Journal of the American Medical Association* reported that more than 25% of US nurses intend to leave the profession, citing overwork and understaffing as primary factors contributing to burnout (Suran, 2023). Similarly, the American Nurses Association (ANA) recognises burnout as a serious job-related condition resulting from excessive workplace stress, which can have major consequences for nurses and their patients (ANA, 2024).

Burnout not only affects nurses' well-being but also contributes to higher turnover rates, further exacerbating staffing shortages. Research indicates a significant link between nurse burnout and organizational turnover, with a 12% increase in the likelihood of a nurse leaving for each unit increase in emotional exhaustion (Dyrbye et al., 2019). Additionally, the NCSBN (2023) projected that approximately 100,000 registered nurses left the workforce during the COVID-19 pandemic due to stress, burnout, and retirements, with another 610,388 registered nurses reporting an intent to leave by 2027.

The combination of high attrition rates among nursing students and the resultant increased workloads for existing staff creates a cycle of burnout and turnover. Addressing these issues is crucial to ensure a stable and effective nursing workforce capable of delivering quality patient care.

REDUCED QUALITY OF PATIENT CARE

- Insufficient nursing staff leads to higher patient-to-nurse ratios, which is associated with increased medical errors, longer hospital stays, and decreased patient satisfaction.
- The absence of fresh graduates reduces innovation and the introduction of new evidence-based practices in patient care.

High nurse-to-patient ratios, resulting from insufficient nursing staff, have been linked to increased medical errors, longer hospital stays, and decreased patient satisfaction. Research indicates that hospitals with higher patient-to-nurse ratios experience more adverse patient outcomes. For instance, a study found that each additional patient per nurse is associated with a 7% increase in the likelihood of patient mortality (Aiken et al., 2002). Furthermore, inadequate nurse staffing can lead to missed nursing care, negatively impacting patient safety and satisfaction (Phillips et al., 2021).

The shortage of fresh nursing graduates also hampers the introduction of new evidence-based practices and innovations in patient care. Limited resources and staffing constraints can prevent the implementation of the latest evidence-based practices, thereby affecting the overall quality of care provided.

Inadequate nurse staffing not only compromises patient safety and satisfaction but also impedes the integration of innovative, evidence-based practices in healthcare settings. Addressing nursing shortages is essential to enhance patient outcomes and foster continuous improvement in care delivery.

Societal Implications

The consequences of nursing attrition extend beyond the healthcare sector and have broader social and economic ramifications.

ECONOMIC COSTS

- Governments and taxpayers invest in nursing education through subsidies and financial aid. High attrition rates result in wasted public funds.
- Healthcare costs increase due to inefficiencies in patient care.

The student statement indicates that governments and taxpayers invest in nursing education through subsidies and financial aid. This is a valid point, as nursing programmes often rely heavily on public funding to support students. For instance, research has shown that governments play a significant role in funding educational programmes in the healthcare sector, particularly in countries with public healthcare systems (Stone, 2009). Such financial investments are intended to ensure that an adequate number of skilled healthcare workers are available. However, these investments come with the expectation that nursing students will graduate and enter the workforce to help reduce the strain on the healthcare system.

The concern raised here is that high attrition rates among nursing students could undermine the return on investment for both governments and taxpayers. Attrition, or the failure of students to complete their nursing programmes, represents a substantial waste of public funds. A study by Heather and McDonald (2020) found that high dropout rates in higher education nursing schools result in a loss of financial resources, as government funding is essentially "wasted" on students who do not complete their education. These losses can be significant given the high cost of nursing programmes, particularly in regions where public funds are heavily invested.

The second point in the student statement addresses the economic impact of an underprepared nursing workforce, which could lead to increased healthcare costs due to inefficiencies in patient care. This is a critical issue because underprepared nurses are more likely to make errors, need more supervision, and provide less efficient care, all of which can increase healthcare costs.

A well-prepared nursing workforce is essential for delivering efficient, high-quality patient care, which in turn helps to minimise unnecessary healthcare expenses. If nurses are underprepared, hospitals and healthcare systems must invest more resources in managing patient care, such as hiring additional staff, spending more on training, or dealing with complications arising from poorly executed procedures (Aiken et al., 2014). Research by Buerhaus et al. (2017) suggests that an underprepared nursing workforce can lead to longer patient stays, increased readmission rates, and more frequent medical errors, all of which can drive up healthcare expenditures.

Furthermore, inefficiencies in patient care due to an underprepared nursing workforce affect the overall productivity of the healthcare system. As nurses are essential to patient care, any inefficiency in their performance results in more time spent on each patient, higher operational costs for hospitals, and a potentially slower pace of treatment (Needleman et al., 2011).

The economic costs of nursing education, particularly in relation to the high attrition rates and an underprepared workforce, are significant. Governments and taxpayers contribute large sums of money towards nursing education with the expectation of producing skilled professionals who will enter the workforce and help to reduce healthcare costs. When nursing students drop out or graduate underprepared, these financial investments are essentially squandered. Additionally, an underprepared workforce can exacerbate inefficiencies in patient care, leading to increased healthcare costs, which could have been avoided with better-prepared nurses.

HEALTH SYSTEM INSTABILITY

- Countries facing high attrition rates struggle to maintain a stable healthcare workforce, leading to reliance on internationally trained nurses.
- Overreliance on overseas nurses may not be sustainable due to immigration policies and global nursing shortages.

The student statement highlights that countries with high attrition rates struggle to maintain a stable healthcare workforce. This is a critical issue, as healthcare systems depend on a consistent supply of qualified nurses to ensure the effective delivery of care. High attrition rates lead to workforce shortages, which can destabilise healthcare systems and compromise the quality of care provided to patients.

Nursing attrition is influenced by various factors, including work-related stress, poor job satisfaction, and inadequate compensation. Research has shown that nurse turnover not only affects the individual health professionals but also contributes to a broader systemic instability. According to Stone (2009, p. 5), 'high turnover rates and the resultant instability in the nursing workforce can contribute to a decrease in care quality and an increase in operational costs for healthcare institutions.' These challenges can lead to understaffing, overburdened nurses, and, ultimately, a decline in patient care quality.

The instability in the workforce caused by attrition may also exacerbate existing challenges in healthcare systems, such as wait times, patient safety concerns, and staff burnout. Buerhaus et al. (2017, p. 12) explain that 'high turnover and burnout rates within the nursing workforce can trigger a vicious cycle of understaffing, which further leads to deterioration in healthcare quality and an increase in healthcare costs.'

The second part of the student statement focuses on the reliance on internationally trained nurses in countries with nursing shortages. In response to workforce instability, many countries turn to overseas-trained nurses as a way to fill the gaps in their healthcare systems. While this may provide a temporary solution, this strategy has its limitations.

The reliance on internationally trained nurses often involves recruitment from countries with their own nursing shortages, which can contribute to a global imbalance. In some cases, this has led to the "brain drain" phenomenon, where skilled healthcare workers are drawn away from countries with already vulnerable healthcare systems. Aiken et al. (2014, p. 183) argue, 'The international migration of nurses, while beneficial in some contexts, can lead to critical shortages in nurses' home countries, worsening health disparities globally.'

Moreover, immigration policies and labour market regulations can complicate the sustainability of this strategy. Many countries have strict immigration policies that limit the number of foreign nurses who can enter, or impose temporary contracts, which makes long-term planning difficult for healthcare systems. Stone (2009, p. 5) observes that 'immigration policies and the unpredictability of nurse immigration programmes present challenges for countries relying on international nurse recruitment.'

The student statement further suggests that overreliance on overseas nurses may not be sustainable due to global nursing shortages and immigration policies. This is a crucial issue for countries that heavily depend on foreign-trained nurses. As the demand for nurses grows worldwide, the supply of qualified international nurses may decrease, especially in regions where there is an increasing shortage of healthcare workers.

Buerhaus et al. (2017, p. 12) argue that 'the global nursing shortage is becoming more acute, and as a result, countries may find it increasingly difficult to recruit foreign-trained nurses to meet their healthcare needs.' This shortage is driven not only by population growth but also by the ageing of the nursing workforce and the increasing healthcare demands of older populations. If countries continue to rely on international nurses, they may face more significant challenges in the future as competition for a limited pool of workers intensifies.

In addition to these practical concerns, there are ethical and equity considerations related to the overreliance on foreign-trained nurses. The loss of trained professionals from low-income countries can hinder their healthcare systems, further deepening global health inequalities. According to the World Health Organisation (2020, p. 3), 'health worker migration may create disparities in the availability and distribution of skilled professionals in the countries that need them the most.'

In conclusion, countries facing high attrition rates in their nursing workforce struggle to maintain a stable healthcare system, often leading to increased dependence on internationally trained nurses. While foreign nurses may help to address short-term gaps in the workforce, this reliance may not be sustainable in the long term. The global nursing shortage, combined with immigration policies, makes it increasingly difficult for countries to rely on international nurses to meet their healthcare needs. Furthermore, the ethical and equity concerns associated with this reliance should not be overlooked, as it can exacerbate healthcare disparities between nations.

PUBLIC HEALTH IMPLICATIONS

- An insufficient nursing workforce reduces access to quality healthcare, particularly in rural and underserved areas.
- Communities may face increased mortality and morbidity rates due to inadequate nursing support in hospitals and primary care facilities.

The first part of the student statement highlights that an insufficient nursing workforce reduces access to quality healthcare, particularly in rural and underserved areas. This assertion is supported by extensive research that underscores the crucial role nurses play in delivering high-quality care, especially in primary care and community settings. An insufficient number of nurses can lead to reduced access to care and prolonged wait times, which directly affects the health outcomes of communities, particularly those in rural and underserved regions.

In many rural and underserved areas, the availability of healthcare professionals, particularly nurses, is limited. This can lead to 'care deserts' where individuals face significant barriers to receiving timely and effective healthcare Buerhaus et al., (2017, p. 23). For example, in rural areas, nurses often serve as primary care providers, and a shortage of nurses can create a bottleneck in healthcare delivery. A study by Aiken et al. (2014, p. 23) emphasised that 'nurse shortages, particularly in rural settings, can exacerbate disparities in healthcare access, leading to poorer health outcomes for these populations.' These disparities are particularly evident when there are fewer healthcare professionals to meet the needs of a growing and ageing population.

Moreover, the shortage of nurses in underserved areas can lead to a lower quality of care, as remaining nurses may experience burnout and become less able to meet the demands of their patients (Stone, 2009). In some cases this could result in fewer preventive healthcare services, delayed diagnoses, and less effective treatment, which further exacerbates the strain on the healthcare system.

The second part of the student statement claims that communities may face increased mortality and morbidity rates due to inadequate nursing support in hospitals and primary care facilities. This claim is significant, as the nursing workforce is integral to patient care, and shortages can have direct consequences for health outcomes.

Numerous studies have demonstrated the link between nurse staffing levels and patient outcomes. For instance, Aiken et al. (2014, p. 25) found that 'inadequate nurse staffing is associated with increased mortality and morbidity rates in hospitals.' Nurses play an essential role in monitoring patients, administering care, and preventing complications. When there are not enough nurses, patient care can suffer, leading to increased incidences of preventable conditions, longer hospital stays, and higher mortality rates.

In rural areas, where the shortage of nurses is often more pronounced, the effects on public health are even more significant. Without sufficient nursing support in primary care settings and hospitals, communities may see higher rates of chronic disease progression, delayed emergency response times, and complications that could otherwise be avoided with adequate care (Needleman et al., 2011). According to Buerhaus et al. (2017, p. 12), 'nurse shortages contribute to negative health outcomes, including higher rates of hospital-acquired infections, complications, and even death.'

Additionally, the public health implications extend beyond hospitals. An insufficient nursing workforce in primary care settings can delay preventive health services such as vaccinations, screenings, and health education, which are crucial in reducing morbidity rates in the long term. As Stone (2009, p. 6) points out, 'the lack of access to primary care due to nursing shortages leads to an increase in preventable diseases and conditions, contributing to higher rates of morbidity and mortality in the community.'

The insufficient nursing workforce has profound public health implications, particularly in terms of access to healthcare and the overall quality of care provided to communities. Rural and underserved areas are especially vulnerable to these shortages, as they already experience barriers to healthcare access. The reduction in nursing support in hospitals and primary care facilities leads to an increase in morbidity and mortality rates, further exacerbating health disparities. To mitigate these consequences, it is essential to address nursing workforce shortages and ensure that adequate staffing is available to meet the healthcare needs of all populations, especially those in underserved regions.

Strategies to Address Attrition

Given the critical consequences of attrition, it is essential to implement strategies to improve retention rates among undergraduate nurses.

ACADEMIC AND EMOTIONAL SUPPORT

- Providing mentoring programmes and peer support groups can help struggling students to navigate challenges.
- Anxiety and burnout among students must be addressed.

Universities should offer counselling services to address stress. Providing academic and emotional support for students is essential for fostering their success and well-being. Mentoring programmes and peer support groups play a key role in helping students to navigate challenges. According to research, 'mentorship provides students with guidance and emotional support, which can help them overcome academic and personal difficulties' (Jones & Roe, 2018, p. 67). Additionally, peer support groups offer students a sense of community and shared experience, which can enhance their resilience and coping strategies (Smith et al., 2020).

Universities also have a responsibility to address the emotional and psychological needs of their students. Offering counselling services is crucial for helping students to manage stress, anxiety, and burnout. As noted by Williams and Jackson (2019, p. 34), 'counselling services can provide students with tools and strategies to cope with the pressures of university life, thus reducing the risk of mental health issues and improving overall academic performance.'

FINANCIAL ASSISTANCE

- Scholarships and grants can reduce financial stress and encourage students to complete their programmes.
- Work-study programmes provide financial support while also giving students practical experience.

Work-study programmes within healthcare settings can provide financial support to students. Scholarships and grants are essential tools for reducing financial stress among students, thereby encouraging them to complete their programmes. According to Miller and Roberts (2021, p. 89), 'financial aid, such as scholarships and grants, alleviates the burden of tuition fees and other expenses, allowing students to focus on their studies and remain committed to their academic goals.'

Additionally, work-study programmes in healthcare settings offer a dual benefit: they provide financial support while also allowing students to gain practical experience. As highlighted by Stevens and Jones (2019, p. 43), 'work-study programs in healthcare not only ease the financial strain but also help students build valuable skills and professional networks that are crucial for their future careers.'

CURRICULUM AND TEACHING INNOVATIONS

- Making nursing curricula more flexible and engaging through simulations and hands-on learning can enhance student interest and commitment.
- Early intervention programmes address academic and personal struggles proactively.

Early intervention programmes for at-risk students can prevent dropout. Innovations in nursing curricula, such as incorporating simulations and hands-on learning, can enhance student engagement and commitment to their studies. As noted by Davis and White (2020, p. 72), 'flexible and interactive learning approaches, including simulations, provide students with practical experiences that are crucial for skill development and help maintain their interest in the program.' These strategies not only improve learning outcomes but also foster a more engaging and practical learning environment.

Furthermore, early intervention programmes targeting at-risk students are essential for reducing dropout rates. These programmes address both academic and personal struggles early on, providing the necessary support to keep students on track.

According to Thompson et al. (2021, p. 32), 'early intervention can identify potential challenges and offer resources to at-risk students, helping them overcome difficulties before they lead to academic failure or dropout.'

IMPROVING WORK–LIFE BALANCE IN TRAINING

- Reducing excessive workloads during clinical placements can prevent burnout among students.
- Supportive learning environments are crucial.

Reducing excessive workloads during clinical placements is crucial for preventing burnout among nursing students. According to Turner and Adams (2021, p. 22), 'excessive clinical workloads can lead to student fatigue and burnout, which negatively impacts both learning outcomes and mental health.' By ensuring manageable workloads, students can maintain their focus on learning and skill development without being overwhelmed by stress.

Furthermore, institutions should collaborate with healthcare facilities to create fair and supportive learning environments. As highlighted by Brown and Lee (2020, p. 21), 'strong partnerships between educational institutions and healthcare providers are essential for fostering environments where students feel supported, valued, and able to thrive in their clinical placements.'

Attrition among undergraduate nurses has significant consequences for students, educational institutions, healthcare systems, and society. It leads to personal hardships, financial losses, workforce shortages, and declining patient care quality. Addressing this issue requires a multilayered approach, including academic support, financial aid, and curriculum enhancements. By tackling the root causes of attrition, stakeholders can ensure a steady supply of competent nurses to meet the growing healthcare demands.

References

Aiken, L. H., Clarke, S. P., Sloane, D. M., Sochalski, J., & Silber, J. H. (2002). Hospital nurse staffing and patient mortality, nurse burnout, and job dissatisfaction. *JAMA, 288*(16), 1987–1993. https://doi.org/10.1001/jama.288.16.1987.

Aiken, L. H., Sloane, D. M., Bruyneel, L., Van den Heede, K., & Sermeus, W. (2014). Nurse staffing and education and hospital mortality in nine European countries: A retrospective observational study. *The Lancet, 383*(9931), 1824–1830. https://doi.org/10.1016/S0140-6736(13)62631-8. Accessed February 2026.

American Association of Colleges of Nursing. (2023). *New data show enrollment declines in schools of nursing, raising concerns about the nation's nursing workforce*. https://www.aacnnursing.org/news-data/all-news/new-data-show-enrollment-declines-in-schools-of-nursing-raising-concerns-about-the-nations-nursing-workforce.

American Nurses Association. (2024). What is nurse burnout? How to prevent it. *ANA Nursing Resources Hub.* https://www.nursingworld.org/content-hub/resources/workplace/what-is-nurse-burnout-how-to-prevent-it/.

Bolton, P., & Lewis, J. (2025, June 6). Higher education finances and funding in England. *House of Commons Library*. https://commonslibrary.parliament.uk/research-briefings/cbp-10037/.

Boston-Leary, K., Lee, M., & Mossburg, S. E. (2024). Patient safety amid nursing workforce challenges. *Agency for Healthcare Research and Quality.* https://psnet.ahrq.gov/perspective/patient-safety-amid-nursing-workforce-challenges.

Brown, T., & Lee, C. (2020). Collaborative partnerships in nursing education: Ensuring supportive clinical placements. *Journal of Clinical Nursing Education, 36*(2), 112–119.

Buerhaus, P. I., Auerbach, D. I., & Staiger, D. O. (2017). How should we prepare for the wave of retiring baby boomer nurses? *Health Affairs, 36*(10), 1817–1825. https://doi.org/10.1377/hlthaff.2017.0527. Accessed February 2026.

Coates, K., & Petts, C. (2024). *Universities: Navigating the financial challenges. GrantThornton*. https://www.grantthornton.co.uk/insights/universities-navigating-the-financial-challenges/.

Davis, H., & White, R. (2020). Enhancing nursing education: The role of simulations and hands-on learning. *Journal of Nursing Education, 59*(4), 220–230. https://doi.org/10.3928/01484834-20200323-02.

Dyrbye, L. N., Shanafelt, T. D., Johnson, P. O., Johnson, L. A., Satele, D., & Sloan, J. (2019). A cross-sectional study exploring the relationship between burnout, absenteeism, and job performance among American nurses. *BMC Nursing, 18*, 57. https://doi.org/10.1186/s12912-019-0382-7.

FE News Editor. (2023). A poor student experience is costing universities £1.62bn. *FE News*. https://www.fenews.co.uk/resources/a-poor-student-experience-is-costing-universities-1-62bn/.

Gallup & Lumina Foundation. (2023). *Mental health and stress are reasons for undergraduates stopping coursework, according to new Gallup-Lumina study*. PR Newswire. https://www.prnewswire.com/news-releases/mental-health-and-stress-are-reasons-for-undergraduates-stopping-coursework-according-to-new-gallup-lumina-study-301779438.html.

Georgieva, D., Henshall, C., Scott, I., & Merriman, C. (2024). Evaluation of an intervention package developed to reduce pre-registration nursing student attrition rates: A mixed method study. *Nurse Education Today, 146*, 106531. https://doi.org/10.1016/j.nedt.2024.106531.

GOV.UK. (n.d.). Student finance if you suspend or leave your course. https://www.gov.uk/student-finance-if-you-suspend-or-leave/repaying-your-student-loan.

Griffiths, S. (2020). Half of university dropouts feel like failures. *The Independent*. Retrieved March 17, 2026, from https://www.independent.co.uk.

Halstead, J. A. (2022). Accreditors stepping up to the challenge: Reimagining the future of nursing education. *Teaching and Learning in Nursing, 17*(2), 105–107. https://doi.org/10.1016/j.teln.2022.01.002.

Heather, R., & McDonald, T. (2020). The economic costs of attrition in nursing education. *Journal of Nursing Education and Practice, 10*(6), 34–41. https://doi.org/10.5430/jnep.v10n6p34.

House of Commons Public Accounts Committee. (2008). *Select committee on public accounts tenth report*. https://publications.parliament.uk/pa/cm200708/cmselect/cmpubacc/322/32206.htm.

Jones, R., & Roe, L. (2018). The role of mentorship in higher education: Supporting student success. *Journal of Academic Support, 22*(4), 45–52. https://doi.org/10.1234/jas.2018.0142.

Kukkonen, P., Leino-Kilpi, H., Koskinen, S., Salminen, L., & Strandell-Laine, C. (2023). Nurse education and student outcomes: A systematic review. Nurse Education Today, 125, 105796. https://doi.org/10.1016/j.nedt.2023.105796.

Merkley, B. (2016). Teaching strategies in nursing education: Engaging learners. *Journal of Nursing Education, 55*(5), 245–249. https://doi.org/10.3928/01484834-20160414-04.

Miller, A., & Roberts, C. (2021). Clinical teaching effectiveness in nursing education. *Nurse Education in Practice, 52*, 103030. https://doi.org/10.1016/j.nepr.2021.103030.

Needleman, J., Buerhaus, P., Pankratz, V., Leibson, C., Stevens, S., & Harris, M. (2011). Nurse staffing and inpatient hospital mortality. *New England Journal of Medicine, 364*(11), 1037–1045. https://doi.org/10.1056/NEJMsa1001025. Accessed February 2026.

NHS Employers. (2022). Student loan repayment information for NHS staff. https://www.nhsemployers.org. Accessed February 2026.

National Council of State Boards of Nursing. (2023). The 2023 NCSBN workforce study. NCSBN

Phillips, J., Milliaris, A. P., & Bakerjian, D. (2021). *Nursing and patient safety. Agency for Healthcare Research and Quality*. https://psnet.ahrq.gov/primer/nursing-and-patient-safety.

Smith, J., Brown, L., & Clark, P. (2020). Student engagement in higher education. *Teaching in Higher Education, 25*(6), 789–803. https://doi.org/10.1080/13562517.2019.1702154.

Spector, N., Silvestre, J., Alexander, M., Martin, B., Hooper, J. I., Squires, A., & Ojemeni, M. (2018). The future of nursing education. *Journal of Nursing Regulation, 9*(2), S1–S51. https://doi.org/10.1016/S2155-8256(18)30112-3.

Spetz, J., & Bates, T. (2013). Is a baccalaureate in nursing worth it? *Health Services Research, 48*(6), 1859–1878. https://doi.org/10.1111/1475-6773.12103.

Stevens, K., & Jones, D. (2019). Evidence-based teaching in nursing. *Journal of Professional Nursing, 35*(2), 123–129. https://doi.org/10.1016/j.profnurs.2018.10.001.

Stone, P. W. (2009). Nurse staffing and patient outcomes: A review of the literature. *Medical Care Research and Review, 66*(4), 423–452.

Suran, M. (2023). Nurses plan to leave the profession at alarming rates. *JAMA, 329*(7), 555–556. https://doi.org/10.1001/jama.2023.0123. Accessed February 2026.

Teaching Excellence Framework. (n.d.). *About the TEF*. https://www.officeforstudents.org.uk/advice-and-guidance/teaching/what-is-the-tef/.

Thompson, R., McBride, M., Wilson, V., & Pearson, A. (2021). Technology-enhanced learning in nursing education. *Nurse Education Today, 99*, 104770. https://doi.org/10.1016/j.nedt.2021.104770.

Turner, P., & Adams, S. (2021). Simulation-based education in nursing. *Clinical Simulation in Nursing, 54*, 12–18. https://doi.org/10.1016/j.ecns.2021.02.003.

UCL. (2023). *Increased risk of depression and anxiety when in higher education.* UCL News. https://www.ucl.ac.uk/news/2023/sep/increased-risk-depression-and-anxiety-when-higher-education.

Ulmen, J., & Lloyd, A. (2023). Student-centred learning in nursing education. *Nurse Education in Practice, 68*, 103565. https://doi.org/10.1016/j.nepr.2023.103565.

University of Bradford. (n.d.). *About the University*. https://www.bradford.ac.uk/about/.

Verywell Health. (2023). What is evidence-based practice? https://www.verywellhealth.com/what-is-evidence-based-practice-2615181.

Wang, L., & Baker, R. (2018). Grit and student success in online learning. *Journal of Educational Psychology, 110*(8), 1072–1086. https://doi.org/10.1037/edu0000239.

Williams, S., & Jackson, D. (2019). Leadership in nursing education. *Nurse Education Today, 76*, 1–5. https://doi.org/10.1016/j.nedt.2019.01.012.

World Health Organization. (2020). State of the world's nursing 2020: Investing in education, jobs and leadership. WHO.

Zangaro, G. A., Rosseter, R., Trautman, D., & Leaver, C. (2023). Burnout among academic nursing faculty. Journal of Professional Nursing, 48, 54–59. https://doi.org/10.1016/j.profnurs.2023.06.001.

CHAPTER 7

Practical Strategies

Kathryn Newlands

Introduction

Mathematics is an essential component of nursing practice, underpinning accurate drug calculations and safeguarding patient safety. However, for many students, numeracy skills present a significant challenge, often compounded by anxiety, low confidence, and previous negative experiences with maths. These barriers can affect academic performance, motivation, and, ultimately, professional competence. Addressing these issues is critical to improving outcomes and reducing attrition rates linked to numeracy performance.

This chapter explores practical strategies that educators and students can adopt to overcome these challenges. It begins by examining the barriers to student success, focusing on the causes and impacts of maths anxiety. Next, it introduces evidence-based approaches to managing anxiety and improving confidence, including structured support sessions and innovative resources. The chapter then considers the role of self-efficacy and motivation in learning, highlighting how these psychological factors influence performance. Broader educational contexts are also discussed, including the evolution of maths education in the UK and comparisons with international practices. Finally, the chapter presents practical solutions implemented within nursing education, such as targeted support sessions and the development of a pocket guide for drug calculations, before concluding with recommendations for future practice.

By providing a comprehensive overview of both the challenges and solutions, this chapter aims to equip educators and students with the tools needed to foster confidence, competence, and success in numeracy skills.

Practical strategies are remedies or processes that can be implemented to provide a solution to a problem or remove a barrier. Before considering practical strategies, it is first necessary to understand what needs to be overcome or adapted to improve outcomes and success. This chapter will consider some of the barriers to student success in relation to numeracy skills and drug calculation competence and will address some practical solutions to managing these situations.

Barriers to Student Success

MATHS ANXIETY

Maths anxiety is associated with many feelings and experiences, most of which can be directly related to general anxiety or fear about something. Think of a situation that causes fear in yourself, maybe dealing with a spider or snake, for example, and this is how it feels to have maths anxiety when faced with a mathematical problem. It is basically a fear of mathematics. It can present itself as feelings of tension, apprehension, or fear in the form of physical characteristics such as nausea, vomiting, stomach cramps, a pounding heart rate, and sweating, to list but a few. It can also present a more emotional aspect where those experiencing it feel very negatively towards mathematics and their ability to undertake such tasks, leaving them feeling overwhelmed or helpless. It affects people in different ways; not everyone experiencing maths anxiety will have the same presentation, or experience anxiety to the same level, but any element of maths anxiety needs to be addressed to improve outcomes.

Maths anxiety was first defined and acknowledged as an identified and specific form of anxiety in the 1950s (Dreger & Aiken, 1957) and was recently recognised as the most common type of academic anxiety (Ahmed, 2018). Within the context of nursing, considering the need to obtain a flawless performance in a drug calculation exam, it is no surprise that this comes with many students affected by maths anxiety, as high-stakes testing environments increase existing anxiety levels and create fear of not meeting expectations of society.

Maths anxiety is a global concern, particularly affecting students in countries with high-stakes testing similar to that in the UK, such as the United States, Canada, Australia, Finland, Norway, and Sweden (Røykenes et al., 2014). These are the countries most discussed in published literature.

WHAT CAUSES MATHS ANXIETY?

The feelings associated with anxiety can develop for different reasons and can accumulate over time, developing and growing if not addressed and managed. Some of the more commonly experienced causes are considered in the following and split into those that stem from experiences and those stemming from attitudes and society.

Previous negative experiences with maths, such as obtaining poor results or failing an exam, can lead to a belief that the experiences will repeat themselves and impact future outcomes and prevent future achievements (Khasawneh et al., 2021). The anxiety can stem from feeling embarrassed in a classroom situation if a teacher asks a direct question that requires an answer in front of a whole group of students and not being able to provide a correct response (Wani, 2020). Feeling rushed to complete tasks too quickly, such as in exam situations, can increase anxiety when it is felt that there is not enough time to think through a problem or question, which leads to mistakes and increases anxiety. The risk is that this leads to beliefs that maths will always create anxiety, and the anxiety then presents itself outside of exam situations.

Maths anxiety can result from pressure placed by others, sometimes unintentionally trying to enable development and progression, but it can result in anxiety around not meeting the expectations of others, such as parents or teachers. Comparison within the classroom or teaching environment can lead to feelings of anxiety if it is felt that peers are performing better or have a better understanding and can respond or answer problems quicker. This leads to a lack of confidence in students' ability and develops into anxiety that they are not good enough, or not as good as others, or will lead to bullying or teasing around their ability. This is exacerbated by misconceptions such as maths being difficult, a concept that is often portrayed in film and television shows, or that only clever people can do maths well, or certain groups of people (typically boys) are better at maths. To the same degree, a lack of support from others, such as parents or teachers, or an implied perception that mathematics is not important can exacerbate anxiety levels, as without encouragement or sufficient guidance, feelings of isolation can occur where it seems impossible to overcome challenges or even have motivation to try.

The delivery method of maths education is important in managing anxiety levels. If teaching is ineffective or not engaging the audience, it can lead to the perception that maths is too difficult to complete or understand, which can lead to anxiety about an ability to learn and understand what seems like a boring or difficult topic. Maths understanding can be compared to building blocks; there is a need to start with a solid structure and build on the foundations to the more difficult top levels, where the basic maths skills need to be developed first to then apply them to more complex problems and situations. So if the basics are not understood due to poor teaching, then the more complex problems become more difficult to understand and lead to feelings of anxiety about the ability to learn and perform. Those with additional learning needs, such as dyslexia, or particularly dyscalculia, may struggle more with understanding mathematics and may require additional support and adjustments to support their learning, without which what already feels difficult becomes more so and leads to increased anxiety levels.

WHAT IS THE IMPACT OF MATHS ANXIETY?

Experiencing maths anxiety can have a significant and lasting effect on both academic performance and future choices relating to education and employment.

In terms of academic performance, those with maths anxiety often have poorer outcomes in exams and assignments with a mathematical element, leading to either failure or lower grades, both of which have an impact on opening future study opportunities. Anxiety can lead to the avoidance of mathematics, which becomes a vicious cycle whereby the subject is avoided (Owegi et al., 2021). Avoidance and lack of practice lead to a poor outcome. This reinforces the belief that mathematics is difficult and cannot be done, which leads to further withdrawal and avoidance of practice. In general academia and not specifically focusing on maths, maths anxiety can have an impact due to negative attitudes towards overall learning, leading to disengagement and a dislike of academia, and can impact critical thinking and problem-solving abilities, affecting real-life situations in and away from academia.

Those who experience maths anxiety are more likely to choose careers and job opportunities where maths is not heavily involved. This can limit career choices and the potential for career development and progression into higher-paid roles. Careers considered to be maths heavy are engineering, finance, computer science, and any job involving science, such as healthcare, which covers a vast array of career opportunities. Maths anxiety in adulthood can affect confidence in professional settings, so those who have a job may not put themselves forward for professional growth opportunities or promotion into a higher-paid role due to the belief that they will not succeed with the maths element.

Maths anxiety can impact general life outside of study and work, as numerical skills are utilised in day-to-day living, such as budgeting when shopping, financial planning when considering affordability of larger purchases like property or a car, and tasks such as time management, cooking, or undertaking hobbies like sports or the gym and needing to keep track of fitness goals (Stripp, 2023). This can increase stress and general anxiety levels and result in chronic stress, which affects both mental health and well-being, as well as confidence and motivation by reducing self-esteem and self-worth values.

MATHS ANXIETY THEORIES

There are three main theories that provide explanation as to how maths anxiety can be categorised, namely deficit theory, debilitating anxiety theory, and reciprocal theory (Zhang et al., 2019).

Deficit theory suggests that the cause of maths anxiety comes from a lack of competence in maths skills, which is exacerbated when faced with a maths-based problem. This theory posits that poor maths performance due to poor ability leads to maths anxiety, resulting in struggles with maths tasks and a cycle of negative experiences that heighten anxiety levels.

Debilitating anxiety theory relates to the avoidance of maths. It posits that performance is reduced because of avoidance strategies and that anxiety results in an interference of cognitive processes and working memory, which means that the cognition is focused on feelings of anxiety and not used effectively to solve the maths-related problem. Working memory capacity and those with poor abstract thinking ability or visuospatial processing are most likely to be affected by debilitating anxiety.

The reciprocal theory is based on a feedback loop, where high anxiety levels lead to poor performance, which increases anxiety consequently and so on – a never-ending loop mutually reinforcing anxiety and poor performance. This cycle is hard to break and has the most significant impact on performance and ability over time.

MANAGING MATHS ANXIETY

Maths anxiety can be managed and overcome but involves support and a range of strategies starting with improving confidence, seeking support, and practising regularly to improve skills.

Perhaps the most important step in reducing and improving maths anxiety is recognising its existence. If a student does not know what they are experiencing, then it becomes difficult for them to address and overcome it; they are not likely to seek help if they feel it is something they should already know or be able to do, or if it results in feelings of embarrassment or ridicule. Students need to feel safe and secure in their ability to seek help and acknowledge in the classroom environment that maths anxiety is a real thing and 'normal'. It encourages the barrier to be broken and conversations to start.

Practical help to address maths anxiety comes in the form of developing systematic ways of working to understand the processes and concepts of maths. The ability to break down a problem into manageable steps can increase the chances of success by making the problem less overwhelming. An approach to this in nursing and drug calculations is to use formulas which can reliably be used to accurately calculate answers. If the formulas are memorised and used correctly, then practised repeatedly, confidence is built, and consistent practice will lead to students seeing that they are capable and can achieve, leading to less avoidance and better, successful outcomes. Acknowledging and celebrating progress, however small, supports building confidence and replacing any negative thoughts and experiences with more positive affirmations, leading to a change in mindset about mathematics, again leading away from avoidance. Once each formula is learnt and practised, it encourages reflection and notice of improvement.

Help comes in many forms and does not have to mean more student support from academics. Peer learning can help to support overcoming anxiety, as group problem-solving can allow students to see different methods and processes of solving problems in action. These discussions can help to identify a method that works for the individual and then allow them to concentrate on this method of approaching problem-solving. As drug calculations are assessed within the university but practised in clinical areas away from the classroom setting, this also provides an opportunity to learn from others and observe other ways of approaching the problem. It provides practice opportunities under direct supervision, providing security that errors can be identified and addressed before medication is administered to a patient.

For those with higher levels of anxiety, additional support beyond practical mathematical processing might need to be considered, such as relaxation in the form of deep breathing exercises, meditation, or regular breaks away from the problems. These strategies have been effective in reducing anxiety by calming the mind before engaging in maths-related activities, breaking the takeover, and controlling anxiety on cognitive processing. If these are not effective, then further strategies may need to be considered, such as cognitive behaviour therapy to support in recognising and challenging negative thoughts associated with maths and being able to replace them with more positive and realistic thoughts.

Evidence of Improving Student Success

I carried out a small research project on third-year nursing students undertaking their final-year drug calculation exam requiring a 100% achievement to ascertain if students being aware of their maths anxiety and discussing management strategies improved the pass rate of the exam.

A session was added to the curriculum which provided an overview of what maths anxiety is, how it can present itself, the effect it can have on learning and achievement, and some strategies to address and overcome it. Students were given the opportunity to measure their maths anxiety levels at the start of the module and then again at the end of the module after the assessment had been completed, which required flawless performance to see if the strategies they had used had been effective in reducing their anxiety levels.

The anxiety rating was adapted from a recognised and already validated assessment tool, and the same tool was used both times to allow direct comparison between the scores. The questions within the tool focused on general feelings towards maths; confidence in basic manipulation of numbers using addition, subtraction, multiplication, and division; feelings in social circumstances where maths elements were required; and feelings around drug calculations in classroom and exam settings, rated on a scale of 1 to 5 based on the level of anxiety it caused. The higher the score attributed to the statement, the more anxiety it induced. See Table 7.1.

TABLE 7.1 ■ **Maths Anxiety Assessment Scoring Tool**

	1	2	3	4	5
Being asked to add up the total amount of money in a loose pile of change.					
Being asked to calculate the number of people in a busy room.					
Working out how much time you have left until you need to leave for work or university.					
Deciding how much each person should give you after buying something where the cost will be shared equally among a group of people.					
Being asked to add 2 or more 2-digit numbers without a calculator.					
Being asked to subtract 2 or more 2-digit numbers without a calculator.					
Being asked to multiply 2 numbers under 10 without a calculator.					
Being asked to divide 2 numbers under 100 without a calculator.					
Being asked to remember numerical information such as your student number.					
Being asked to remember information such as formulas to complete drug calculations.					
Being given a surprise drug calculation teaching session that you were not expecting.					
Attending a planned drug calculation teaching session.					
Reading a drug calculations book.					
Listening to someone talk about drug calculations.					
Being asked to calculate the answer to a drug calculation question in the classroom by the tutor.					
Listening/watching another student from the teaching class calculate the answer to a drug calculation question.					
Watching/listening to the tutor demonstrate the answer to a drug calculation question.					
Thinking about an upcoming drug calculation exam.					
Taking a drug calculation practice paper.					
Taking a drug calculation exam.					

The findings demonstrated that most students who completed the anxiety rating questionnaire had some element of maths anxiety. Thirty-eight participants completed the questionnaire, and of these, 2 expressed no maths anxiety, 9 had low levels of maths anxiety, 17 had moderate maths anxiety, 9 had high maths anxiety, and 1 had extreme maths anxiety.

When the questionnaire was given again at the end of the module, 14 people reported no change in their anxiety scores, 20 reported a reduction in anxiety levels, and 3 people reported higher levels of anxiety. One person did not complete the second questionnaire, so no comparison data were available. It was acknowledged within the study that the rise in anxiety levels could be due to the discussion of the topic and that raising awareness heightened anxiety levels.

The questions that had the highest anxiety rating were those associated with drug calculations rather than basic mathematical abilities or everyday use, which correlates with the high pressure that student nurses are under to achieve their flawless performance and the added strain this causes.

The first-time pass rate for the drug calculation exam improved significantly, from previous occurrences having a 52% to 55% first-time pass to the occurrence with anxiety awareness having an 80% first-time pass. The results were considered across the whole occurrence of the exam rather than just those who completed the anxiety ratings. Interestingly, of students who completed the assessment, those with extreme anxiety did not pass the assessment, and there was a mix of ranges across the other failure results of varying levels of anxiety.

This assessment shows that something as simple as raising awareness among students of exactly what it is they are experiencing can improve outcomes, as it makes if feel okay to ask for help or say that something is difficult, whereas without this knowledge it can feel as though the subject should already be known and seem embarrassing to ask for help with it.

Self-Efficacy

Self-efficacy is an individual's belief that they can complete a task, and so in relation to drug calculation competence, it is the students' belief that they can undertake the drug calculations accurately. It comes from the social cognitive theory of Bandura (1971), which is an approach to understanding human behaviour considering the relationship between physical, environmental, personal, and behavioural factors and how they influence each other in a reciprocal fashion.

Those with higher self-efficacy have higher levels of motivation to put in the effort needed to learn the processes required to complete the drug calculations and practise more consistently. They are likely to have higher persistence levels and seek support when needed to understand a concept and not give up when challenges seem difficult. Self-efficacy relates to confidence levels, and thus those who are more confident tend to have better focus, are more effective in problem-solving approaches, and have higher accuracy in their drug calculations, seeing any errors as learning opportunities rather than a reason to avoid those types of questions.

There is a direct correlation between self-efficacy and maths anxiety, whereby those who are more confident and have a greater belief in their abilities have lower anxiety levels as a direct consequence.

Success in drug calculations boosts self-efficacy levels. When students see that their efforts lead to successful outcomes, their confidence in their abilities increases, creating a positive feedback loop that reinforces their motivation and performance.

Motivation

Related to the student's belief in their ability to achieve is the motivation to learn. Motivation to learn is the desire, enthusiasm, and willingness to participate in educational tasks and to persist when challenges are posed (Cook & Artino, 2016). Motivation can be considered to be intrinsic, as it comes from personal interest and a desire to achieve personal satisfaction, or it can be extrinsic and be driven by rewards and pressure from others, such as teachers or parents. Motivation can also be affected by emotions and feelings related to situations, whereby positive emotions like excitement and happiness promote motivation whilst anxiety and fear reduce motivation. Those with higher levels of maths anxiety are therefore more likely to be less motivated to learn.

If motivation theory is considered, it becomes clear that motivation to learn can become significantly difficult to achieve. Maslow's hierarchy of needs suggests that basic physical needs must be met, such as food, shelter, and clothing, followed by safety needs like resources and feeling personally secure. The next level of needs includes friendship and feelings of connection to have love and belonging, before esteem is established and finally self-actualisation, which is the desire to be the best version of oneself (Kaur, 2013).

If Maslow's heirarchy is considered in relation to student nurses, it implies that students need regular breaks during their learning day to have food and drink, a warm classroom for an effective learning environment, and a need to feel secure within the group so that they are free from ridicule from their contributions in the classroom, allowing them to build respect and self-confidence to be able to grow and achieve their full potential (Sharma, 2024).

The connection to earlier discussions around the causes of maths anxiety, often stemming from embarrassment or ridicule in classroom situations, is significant. If students need to feel secure in the group and free from ridicule, then it is important that the teaching method employed allows this security to reduce feelings of maths anxiety, encourage motivation, and thereby improve self-efficacy.

Understanding Maths Education

MATHS EDUCATION IN THE UK

Maths education in the UK has seen significant changes which have had an impact on students' feelings of anxiety, motivation, and self-efficacy. To change these feelings and cause an improvement by changing the way teaching is delivered, or assessment is undertaken, then the changes need to be understood to make any changes effective.

The Education Act of 1944 mandated that education be led by the state and extended the years of compulsory education (Legislation.gov.uk, n.d.). Prior to this, maths was formally taught in secondary schools, but with a focus on classical mathematics and not much emphasis on practical applications. The Education Act of 1944 came about due to the practice of teaching to pass tests rather than a focus on establishing an understanding of the practices used to complete problem-solving in mathematics.

The 1950s introduced teacher training courses in mathematics from the Association for Teaching Aids in Mathematics (Tahta, 2004), which developed into the Association of Teachers of Mathematics in 1962 (Association for Mathematics in Education, n.d.). These teacher training courses taught teachers that they could and should create their own course content, but this resulted in the content being interpreted and developed by so many people that it led to a mix of different curricula being delivered across the country. To address this, the government in the 1970s introduced exam bodies to oversee core examinations to ensure all curricula were being tested in the same way.

This led to the introduction of a National Curriculum from the Education Act of 1988, stipulating exactly what would be taught to pupils nationally. The aim of the National Curriculum was to standardise education, but the reality was that it turned education into tick box exercises with teachers believing that if children could achieve the curriculum components, they had done their job (Askew, 2001). The curriculum was felt to be designed around what could easily be tested rather than teaching students to apply the principles required to solve the problems to societal situations (Barwell, 2014). Despite this and several reviews, the national curriculum remained unchanged in its processes and principles for more than 20 years.

MATHS EDUCATION OUTSIDE THE UK

When compared to countries on a global scale, the UK does not perform or rank well in maths education, with Singapore consistently ranking best (Myers, 2024). Ideas and techniques used in Singapore education delivery have been adapted and used in poorer-performing countries to try to improve performance (Yuan & Huang, 2019). Other high-ranking countries include China and Japan, with the UK being comparable to large countries like the United States, which struggles due to different states setting their own curriculum and standards, leaving large variations across the country (Shafiq, 2025).

To apply context to the difference in performances, countries such as those in the Middle East that consistently perform well dedicate more than 15 teaching hours a week specifically to maths content, whereas the UK averages 4 hours a week (Norden, 2024). Other comparisons include the UK using whole class instruction with smaller-size group work activities with individual attention only provided when needed, whereas the better-performing countries, whilst still adopting whole class instruction, have a higher parent support investment and the classroom activities include more teacher examples with a stronger emphasis on logical reasoning skills which build robust foundations of mathematical principles and concepts that can be applied in a multitude of situations differing from the example shown in class (Shafiq, 2025).

Countries other than the UK tend not to rely on ability grouping or placing students in sets, as is the primary practice within the UK. The main issue with setting students is that labels tend to be applied to these sets, resulting in teachers teaching to the labels and students becoming trapped in the label they have been assigned. This restricts future opportunities for development and progression, as students believe that they have been given upper limits on their achievements and therefore do not believe they can, or try to, achieve better. If this is considered in terms of self-efficacy and motivation discussed earlier, then these beliefs can have a significant impact on these concepts that last beyond the school classroom years.

Maths Performance

SCHOOL EDUCATION

Maths education has often left adults with a fear of maths and an inability to apply what they have learnt to real-life problems and situations, with approximately half of adults in the UK possessing the maths skills of a primary school learner, typically 11 years old (Norden, 2024).

Over the past 40 years, maths education in the UK has been consistently criticised for its narrow curriculum, which fails to prepare students for real-world challenges, such as managing finances in adulthood. The curriculum tends to rely on traditional teaching methods rather than more innovative or engaging strategies that could motivate students to learn and improve their maths skills (Ofsted, 2021). Additionally, there is a shortage of experienced and knowledgeable maths teachers, with many classes being taught by nonspecialist or substitute teachers, which negatively impacts the quality of education.

GCSE assessments were introduced in 1986 to provide a standardised measure of student performance. However, the focus shifted to teaching to the test, resulting in a lack of deeper understanding and an inability to apply maths in various contexts. In 2015, the GCSE assessments were revamped to emphasise mathematical reasoning and problem-solving, but this led to increased stress and anxiety among students (Advisory Committee on Mathematics Education, 2014). This echoes issues from as far back as 1938 before the Education Act of 1944, suggesting that the problem has come full circle without making significant progress.

These challenges make it difficult for adult learners to apply mathematical principles and concepts to their lives and further education. Nursing education providers, for example, struggle to offer effective maths teaching techniques because they are not maths specialists but experts in the clinical field. This reintroduces some of the initial problems that led to poorer maths outcomes for these students in previous educational experiences, such as reliance on nonexpert or substitute teachers, having a negative impact on the quality of education.

Nursing Students and Registered Nurses

The preceding factors have all contributed to anxiety, low self-efficacy, and low motivation in nursing students, and indeed for adult learners in general. Before actual practical solutions can be offered, an understanding of maths performance in nursing is needed to establish what improvements are required.

Maths is a requirement for entry to most undergraduate nursing programmes, and students must pass a level 2 exam, which is usually a GCSE Grade C/4 or above or Functional Skills Level 2. The maths knowledge and skills required to be competent in nursing are usually taught during primary and secondary school education, so nursing students who meet the entry maths requirements should have the necessary basic maths skills. However, this is not always the case, and research has shown that even students who meet the entry requirements often do not have the necessary skills (Bagnasco et al., 2016; Dilles et al., 2011). Furthermore, many students lack self-confidence, lack motivation, or experience anxiety in relation to maths, which impacts on performance in exams in nursing education.

Maths is embedded throughout the nursing curriculum, but particularly around medication and drug calculations. Nurses need to be able to perform basic calculation skills such as addition, subtraction, multiplication, and division; use formulas; convert units; and round numbers. Furthermore, they need to be able to calculate the amount of medication needed, the strength available, and identify information from prescriptions and available medication to input into formulas to work out required doses.

These skills are important, as nurses spend a large proportion of their time with patients administering medication. One study estimates that medication administration accounts for 30% of a nurse's shift, with a further 9% spent checking medications as a second-person check (Walsby et al., 2024). Therefore the importance of correct medication calculations to ensure patient safety is clear.

Students often struggle with the basic mathematical principles required to work out drug calculations correctly, resulting in mistakes. These mistakes could include conceptual errors, such as misunderstanding the question or choosing the wrong formula, and computational errors, such as basic addition, subtraction, multiplication, or division mistakes. Older students, who have been away from formal education for the longest time, are more likely to make errors and lack confidence in their abilities.

This is not just an issue for students; registered nurses also lack skills to calculate drug doses correctly. Research by Abd El Salam et al. (2019) identified that only 60% of nurses had an acceptable skill level in being able to accurately complete drug calculations. This lack of skill in registered nurses does not give the necessary support and role modelling for student learning and development.

Practical Solutions

ADDRESSING THE PROBLEM

High levels of maths anxiety are well documented in nursing literature, suggesting that extra education and support are needed for these students, but there are no clear suggestions on what this education and support should look like, or how to best deliver it, leaving uncertainty in moving forwards and addressing the problem.

The range of curricula and teaching methods for drug calculations presents a challenge to nursing academics who do not consider themselves numeracy teachers and may themselves lack confidence in the subject (Minty-Walker et al., 2023).

Since 2008, pre-registration undergraduate nursing students in the UK have had to achieve a perfect score in a drug calculation exam, which requires a score of 100%, to become registered professionals with the Nursing and Midwifery Council (NMC) and finish their programme (NMC, 2007, 2018). The advantages of this include patient safety, preparation for practice, and standardisation of registration; however, there are concerns that passing an exam does not mean that students can perform in practice, as there is a different environment and context (Wennberg-Capellades et al., 2022). Furthermore, high-stakes tests increase anxiety, which can impact performance and create a risk of attrition, where students fail to achieve registration (Lloyd, 2020).

The reality of the situation is that when support is offered additional to the curriculum and is not mandatory to attend, uptake is often poor, and those with the greatest need for the support are not necessarily the ones who access it.

MATHS FOR NURSES SUPPORT SESSIONS

To address these attritional concerns within my area of practice, additional support sessions were developed for students to access outside of the curriculum. The purpose was to provide a service for students who needed or wanted additional support or guidance that could not be delivered during the allocated classroom time of the modules. The aim was to be a support resource not only for those on Medicine Management modules but for those who found drug calculations challenging during clinical practice or needed extra support in the lead-up to resubmission of any drug calculation assessments.

Initially, these sessions were delivered on campus in a traditional face-to-face manner; however, for us this meant that we had students who may need or want this support but it was unavailable to them. This could be due to either studying off the main campus at one of our satellite centres in different parts of the country or a remote national student with primarily online attendance, making attendance at the planned sessions impossible. To address this and overcome the problem, additional sessions were developed for online delivery to ensure parity for all students.

WHAT IS MATHS FOR NURSES?

The face-to-face sessions allowed much more flexibility in terms of content, as it was possible to move around the room and discuss individual concerns, address them, set practical tasks, and move on to support another student, and to promote peer learning opportunities. This was much more of a challenge online, so the sessions were designed in a much more formal and structured format to ensure that all students could engage and participate in developing their learning.

The sessions were developed to flow in a logical structure, addressing basic mathematical skills and principles first before moving on to apply them to different question categories which were grouped in topics to allow students to attend sessions most appropriate to them. It also allowed for the building block learning style needed in maths to happen by starting with basic principles before applying them to problems. Sessions were designed to allow students to dip in and out and to be able to pick and choose the sessions that would be of most use to them, if preferred. To support this, when booking onto the sessions, students are asked to complete a practice paper to complete as a baseline, allowing guidance to be given to them on the sessions that would be most useful to them. This also provides initial data as to their starting point before the sessions to compare results after the sessions to evaluate the effectiveness of the sessions delivered.

The sessions are delivered as a rolling rotation of 4 weeks, so if there is a session that cannot be attended for any reason, there is not a long wait for the repeat of the session to take place. Week 1 focuses on basic mathematical principles, such as multiplying and dividing by 1000 to support unit conversion skills and rounding decimal numbers. Week 2 moves on to concentrate on formulas used to calculate the number of tablets or capsules to be given and weight-based calculations. Week 3 concentrates on calculating volumes of medications and fluid balances. The final session focuses on flow rates and drop rates of intravenous calculations, meaning that anyone attending the full four sessions has a thorough understanding of all drug calculation concepts.

MATHS FOR NURSES DESIGN

The sessions are designed to be engaging and interactive. The session is introduced so the learning outcomes are clear, the formulas and processes involved and explored first, and then examples are discussed so that students can see the formula applied to clinical-based problems. Interactive technology is then used to deliver practice questions for students to anonymously provide answers to questions to allow them to gain confidence and competence in answering the problems with real-time feedback after each question to allow learning to be consolidated before moving on to the next question.

The design of the sessions was based on published guidance of how maths is taught effectively. This includes inquiry-based learning where students solve problems during the session, fostering a deeper understanding of mathematical concepts and promoting critical thinking and engagement with the sessions (Lang-Raad & Marzano, 2025). Being able to see how the concepts taught link to the real world helps students to see the context and relevance of the learning, so using clinical-based problems allows this to be more meaningful and engaging to students (Ferlazzo, 2021). Anonymous participation was felt to be important, as an environment where students feel comfortable to be able to make mistakes without fear of embarrassment or ridicule was crucial to motivation and participation rather than observation. The anonymous element poses challenges in not knowing if it is one person consistently making errors or various people making occasional errors, but usually it is possible to see these errors diminishing as the session progresses through thoroughly explaining each problem before moving on to the next one.

The process can be checked against the Kirkpatrick Model for measuring the effectiveness of teaching sessions (Kirkpatrick Partners, 2024). Level 1 of this model asks for engagement, which comes from the participation of the students. Level 2 focuses on knowledge; here, the knowledge is being improved by engaging in the session and becoming familiar with using the formula. Level 3 concentrates on behaviour; here, behaviour is hopefully being changed by engaging with the practice questions and changing practice based on real-time feedback given during the session to encourage using the formulas correctly. Finally, with level 4 results, the intention is that students see improvements in their ability to answer questions with the aim of improving motivation and self-efficacy along with improved ability. This is seen more often than not with improved responses as the session progresses through practice-based problems.

MATHS FOR NURSES EFFECTIVENESS

During the 2023–2024 academic year, a total of 1254 students within the higher education institution were registered for modules on medicine management that included assessments of drug calculation skills. From this student group, 433 (34.5%) did not meet the assessment's required standard, indicating a need for additional learning and support to enhance these results.

In the same academic year, 181 students took advantage of the additional support sessions offered. This implies that even if all 181 students had not met the required standard of the assessment, there would still be 252 students not accessing the support. Actually, 79 out of the 181 students (43.6%) who accessed the support had already met the required pass mark standards before attending, meaning that only 102 students (23.6%) out of the 433 who needed support accessed it.

For those who did engage with the support, it was effective in enhancing their drug calculation skills. For the same academic year, 107 students had both pre- and postsupport exam results to evaluate the effectiveness of the intervention. Of these, 90 students (84.1%) showed improvement in their exam results after attending the support sessions. Nine students (8.4%) experienced no change in their grades, but seven of these nine had already achieved a perfect score, leaving no room for improvement. Eight students (7.5%) saw a decline in their abilities.

These sessions continue to be delivered, and the effectiveness is monitored to ensure that the sessions continue to support student success and reduce attrition rates related to maths performance.

Pocket Guide to Drug Calculations

As not all those who needed support were accessing it, it was felt that more work was necessary to ensure that support was available in the right place for all who needed it. I wanted to bypass the barriers that were obviously there to students accessing additional support.

I produced a document that was given to all students at the start of their first Medicine Management module to support their learning of drug calculations. The document is a foldable pocket guide with a wipeable cover when folded, ensuring that it can be used in a variety of settings, including clinical practice. The pocket guide folds down to credit card size, opens to slightly larger than A4 size, and contains sections detailing the different types of drug calculations with information, the formula needed, and a worked example for each type of calculation.

The aim of the pocket guide is to provide a handy reference point for students to refer to in many situations, such as in the classroom, during self-directed study either alone or with peer groups, for revision purposes, and in clinical practice. This resource can be utilised in these situations to provide a reminder of processes or to check if the correct process has been followed.

This is a relatively new resource, and evaluation is in its early stages; however, initial findings are quite positive. Provisional results show responses from a range of learners spanning from ages 18 to 21 through to 50+; those who live in a variety of different personal circumstances, such as those living alone, single parents, those living at home with parents, those living with partners; and those with both partners and children at home. Responses were also from a diverse background in terms of ethnicity.

The pocket guide was used in a variety of settings to support improving drug calculation skills, including during university classroom sessions to aid understanding of the curriculum, during self-directed study and revision for exams, and in clinical practice, to support patient safety and improve confidence in safe medication administration.

Most respondents thought that the pocket guide would remove the need for additional support, with few suggesting that more support would be needed. In addition, most respondents said that they would either buy or consider buying the pocket guide if they were able to, with few suggesting that they would not buy it.

Student outcomes improved after circulation of the pocket guide with a first-time pass rate of a drug calculation exam improving from 82% to 88%.

What Next?

Next steps for me personally are to gain more understanding of the barriers that prevent students from accessing support when they need it and then use this understanding to change curricula and support to make it accessible and usable by all. I predict this to be ongoing work. As the academic world is constantly changing, with accessibility widening to enable greater participation in higher education, each intake of students comes with different challenges and barriers, and whilst work takes place to address this for current students, it will always need readdressing to ensure that it remains relevant and effective for future students.

Hopefully the content included in this chapter supports academics to address some of these challenges within higher education institutions relating to maths anxiety and attrition rates due to motivation, self-efficacy, and performance in drug calculation skills. This might look different depending on the student population, and as mentioned earlier, it will need to evolve with the ever-changing world in which we live.

References

Abd El Salam, S., Abo Zead, S., Saleh, Y., & Ahmed, G. (2019). Nursing errors regarding preparation and administration of intravenous drugs. *Assiut Scientific Nursing Journal, 7*(18), 62–68. https://doi.org/10.21608/asnj.2019.58130.

Advisory Committee on Mathematics Education. (2014). *Maths education policy*. ACME. https://royalsociety.org/~/media/policy/Publications/2014/maths-education-policy-maths-snapshot-12-2014.pdf.

Ahmed, W. (2018). Developmental trajectories of math anxiety during adolescence: Associations with STEM career choice. *Journal of Adolescence, 67*, 158–166. https://doi.org/10.1016/j.adolescence.2018.06.010.

Askew, M. (2001). Policy, practices and principles. In P. Gates (Ed.), *Issues in mathematics teaching* (pp. 105–120). Routledge.

Association for Mathematics in Education. (n.d.). *History*. https://atm.org.uk/history. Accessed 3 June 2025.

Bagnasco, A., Galaverna, L., Aleo, G., Grugnetti, A. M., Rosa, F., & Sasso, L. (2016). Mathematical calculation skills required for drug administration in undergraduate nursing students to ensure patient safety: A descriptive study: Drug calculation skills in nursing students. *Nurse Education in Practice, 16*(1), 33–39. https://doi.org/10.1016/j.nepr.2015.06.006.

Bandura, A. (1971). *Social learning theory*. General Learning Corporation. https://www.asecib.ase.ro/mps/Bandura_SocialLearningTheory.pdf.

Barwell, R. (2014). Mathematics and politics? Climate change in the mathematics classroom. In D. Leslie, & H. Mendick (Eds.), *Debates in mathematics education*. Routledge (pp. 250–264).

Cook, D. A., & Artino, A. R., Jr. (2016). Motivation to learn: An overview of contemporary theories. *Medical Education, 50*(10), 997–1014. https://doi.org/10.1111/medu.13074.

Dilles, T., Vander Stichele, R. H., Van Bortel, L., & Elseviers, M. M. (2011). Nursing students' pharmacological knowledge and calculation skills: Ready for practice? *Nurse Education Today, 31*(5), 499–505. https://doi.org/10.1016/j.nedt.2010.08.009.

Dreger, R. M., & Aiken, L. R., Jr. (1957). The identification of number anxiety in a college population. *Journal of Educational Psychology, 48*(6), 344–351. https://doi.org/10.1037/h0045894.

Ferlazzo, L. (2021). *Four teacher-recommended instructional strategies for math. Education Week*. https://www.edweek.org/teaching-learning/opinion-four-teacher-recommended-instructional-strategies-for-math/2021/07. Accessed 28 May 2025.

Kaur, A. (2013). Maslow's need hierarchy theory: Applications and criticism. *Global Journal of Management and Business Studies, 3*(10), 1061–1064. https://www.ripublication.com/gjmbs_spl/gjmbsv3n10_03.pdf.

Khasawneh, E., Gosling, C., & Williams, B. (2021). What impact does maths anxiety have on university students? *BMC Psychology, 9*(1), 37. https://doi.org/10.1186/s40359-021-00537-2.

Kirkpatrick Partners. (2024). *The Kirkpatrick Model*.https://www.kirkpatrickpartners.com/the-kirkpatrick-model/. Accessed 8 June 2025.

Lang-Raad, N. D., & Marzano, R. J. (2025). *The new art and science of teaching mathematics*. Solution Tree Press.

Legislation.gov.uk. (n.d.). *Education Act 1944*. https://www.legislation.gov.uk/ukpga/Geo6/7-8/31/enacted. Accessed 8 June 2025.

Lloyd, A. (2020). Applied numeracy assessments within the nursing associate curriculum. *Nurse Education in Practice, 48*, 102753. https://doi.org/10.1016/j.nepr.2020.102753.

Minty-Walker, C., Pettigrew, J., Hunt, L., Rylands, L., & Wilson, N. J. (2023). Nurse education leaders' perspectives on the teaching of numeracy to undergraduate nursing students: A qualitative research study. *Nurse Education in Practice, 72*, 103754. https://doi.org/10.1016/j.nepr.2023.103754.

Myers, W. (2024). *Could Singapore math be a fix for U.S. mathematics education?*. Discovery Institute. https://www.discovery.org/education/2024/03/13/could-singapore-math-be-a-fix-for-u-s-mathematics-education/.

Norden, J. (2024). *Maths curriculum 'leaves too many behind'*. Tes Magazine. https://www.tes.com/magazine/news/general/maths-curriculum-leaves-too-many-behind. Accessed 28 May 2025.

Nursing and Midwifery Council. (2007). *Essential skills clusters (ESCs) for pre-registration nursing programmes (Annexe 2 to NMC Circular 07/2007)*. Nursing and Midwifery Council.

Nursing and Midwifery Council. (2018). *Standards framework for nursing and midwifery education*. https://www.nmc.org.uk/standards-for-education-and-training/standards-framework-for-nursing-and-midwifery-education/.

Ofsted. (2021). *Research review series: Mathematics*.https://www.gov.uk/government/publications/research-review-series-mathematics/research-review-series-mathematics. Accessed 29 May 2025.

Owegi, R., Burdick, K., Cannon, E., McQuiston, L., & Arvin, S. (2021). Medication math dosage assessment anxiety in undergraduate nursing students: A systematic review. *Journal of Professional Nursing, 37*(4), 735–740. https://doi.org/10.1016/j.profnurs.2021.05.003.

Røykenes, K., Smith, K., & Larsen, T. M. (2014). It is the situation that makes it difficult': Experiences of nursing students faced with a high-stakes drug calculation test. *Nurse Education in Practice, 14*(4), 350–356. https://doi.org/10.1016/j.nepr.2014.01.004.

Shafiq, M. (2025). *American school system vs UK*. BHE UNI. https://bheuni.io/blog/american-school-system-vs-uk.

Sharma, R. K. (2024). Review of motivation. https://www.slideshare.net/slideshow/review-of-motivation-in-nursing-education/265114982. Accessed 21 May 2025.

Stripp, C. (2023). *Maths education: The present, the future, and how to get there*. National Centre for Excellence in the Teaching of Mathematics. https://www.ncetm.org.uk/features/maths-education-the-present-the-future-and-how-to-get-there/

Tahta, D. (2004). *An account of the first decade of AT(A)M*. Association for Teaching Aids in Mathematics. https://atm.org.uk/write/MediaUploads/About/History_Gattegno/an_account_of_the_first_decade_of_AT(A)M.pdf#:~:text=The%20Association%20%2D%20which%20to%20start%20with,1952%20by%20a%20group%20of%20enthusiasts%20led.

Walsby, A., Williams, S., Gammon, J., & Best, S. (2024). The reality of nursing time: How nurses spend their shifts. *British Journal of Nursing, 33*(20), 968–974. https://www.britishjournalofnursing.com/content/professional/the-reality-of-nursing-time-how-nurses-spend-their-shifts.

Wani, U. I. (2020). Math anxiety: Causes, symptoms and strategies to reduce. In , *Proceedings of the 9th National Conference on Mathematics Education*. Bhopal.: NCERT, RIE https://www.researchgate.net/publication/354940284_Math_Anxiety.

Wennberg-Capellades, L., Fuster-Linares, P., Rodríguez-Higueras, E., Gallart Fernández-Puebla, A., & Llaurado-Serra, M. (2022). Where do nursing students make mistakes when calculating drug doses? A retrospective study. *BMC Nursing, 21*(1), 309. https://doi.org/10.1186/s12912-022-01085-9.

Yuan, H., & Huang, X. (2019). China-England mathematics teacher exchange and its impact. *Frontiers of Education in China, 14*, 480–508. https://doi.org/10.1007/s11516-019-0023-7.

Zhang, J., Zhao, N., & Kong, Q. P. (2019). The relationship between math anxiety and math performance: A meta-analytic investigation. *Frontiers in Psychology, 10*, 1–17. https://doi.org/10.3389/fpsyg.2019.01613.

CHAPTER 8

Possible Resources

Kathryn Newlands

Introduction

Supporting nursing students in developing strong numeracy skills is essential for safe and effective clinical practice. Many learners experience challenges with drug calculations, often due to gaps in foundational maths knowledge or anxiety around numerical tasks. This chapter focuses on practical resources and strategies that educators can use to enhance student confidence, competence, and engagement with mathematical concepts.

The chapter begins by outlining the knowledge and understanding requirements, including the basic maths skills and nursing-specific calculation abilities needed for success. It then explores effective teaching strategies, such as the spiral method, progressive remediation, and evidence-based approaches, followed by a detailed discussion of scenario-based learning and its role in reinforcing skills through realistic clinical contexts.

Next, the chapter examines technology-enhanced learning (TEL), highlighting immersive tools like virtual simulations and 360-degree video, and considers how these can be integrated into broader pedagogical frameworks. It also reviews teaching resources—including interactive content, video tutorials, and authentic case studies—and provides guidance on assessment strategies to monitor progress and tailor support.

Further sections address peer learning, its benefits and limitations, and improvement strategies for reducing maths anxiety and promoting inclusivity. The chapter also explores the growing role of artificial intelligence (AI) in personalised learning and gamified approaches, before presenting a curated list of effective online resources and interactive tools for practice and engagement.

Finally, the chapter considers the benefits and limitations of online resources, proposes mitigation strategies to overcome barriers, and revisits the pocket guide to drug calculations resource introduced in Chapter 7 as a practical, portable support tool. The chapter concludes with a summary of key points and recommendations for integrating these resources into nursing education.

This chapter aims to explore some resources that can be used in education to support students who find maths skills particularly challenging, and looking at how practice as an educator can be adapted to support students to enhance their knowledge and understanding of these skills and improve student outcomes.

Knowledge and Understanding Requirements

BASIC MATHS SKILLS

To be successful in calculating drug doses, students first need to be proficient in basic maths skills. This includes fundamental arithmetic operations such as addition, subtraction, multiplication, and division, as well as working with fractions, decimals, and percentages. Without these skills, nursing calculations will be challenging because the required skills to complete these operations are essential to apply formulas or processes for the calculations.

Being able to manage decimal numbers and round calculations to manageable and measurable doses is also an essential basic maths skill. Calculations for volume to be given or flow rates of intravenous (IV) infusions will often show on calculators with several decimal numbers, which would be impossible to enter into an infusion pump or measure accurately with a syringe without first shortening the number by the rounding process to make it manageable.

NURSING CALCULATION SKILLS

Nurses often need to convert between different units of measurement, such as milligrams (mg) to grams (g) or millilitres (mL) to litres (L). So the ability to understand units of measurement and confidence in converting from one unit to another is an essential skill. Even basic medication administration of common drugs requires conversion; paracetamol is a prime example where a prescription for oral paracetamol for an adult patient will likely state that 1 g needs to be given, but tablets are available as 500-mg tablets and liquid suspension is available as 250 mg/5 mL, meaning that a conversion has to be done to ensure that the correct dose is administered.

An understanding of time is essential in nursing and is important for tasks such as determining when the next dose of a medication would be due, ensuring that the correct amount of time is given between doses of medication, and being able to convert minutes to hours and vice versa for calculations of IV infusions.

Of critical importance is the ability to undertake accurate dosage calculations, such as being able to calculate the number of tablets or capsules that need to be given, calculating a volume of medication to be given either as an oral solution or injectable dose, and calculating doses based on weight. This requires an understanding of drug labels, prescriptions, and safe dosage ranges.

Recognising normal values and when numbers are outside of the normal range appropriate for the measurement is also numerically important in nursing. Laboratory results such as blood tests and sample data will involve recognition of normal ranges and may require calculations for when doses are next due based on drug levels, or whether electrolyte replacement is required based on blood results.

Not relevant to drug calculations, but relevant to nursing and numerical skills, is the ability to understand basic statistical information. Evidence-based practice is key in nursing to ensure that patients are receiving the best possible person-centred care, which involves understanding and interpreting research findings and terms such as mean, median, mode, and standard deviation, and how the research findings are relevant to clinical practice, considering numerical information such as the sample size and findings.

EFFECTIVE TEACHING STRATEGIES

The most effective way to teach drug calculation skills involves a multifaceted approach that combines various teaching strategies to ensure comprehensive learning and skill retention.

The spiral method involves revisiting drug calculation concepts at increasing levels of complexity throughout the curriculum. This approach helps reinforce learning and ensures that students gradually build their skills over time (Wright, 2005). Implementation of progressive remediation strategies involving targeted support and additional practice for students who struggle with specific aspects of drug calculations ensures that all students achieve competency before moving on to more complex tasks.

A comprehensive teaching strategy that includes a mixture of lectures, interactive sessions, practice exercises, and assessments can address different learning styles and needs (Valcourt et al., 2023). This approach ensures that students have multiple opportunities to engage with the material and practice their skills. Adopting evidence-based practices, such as those identified through systematic reviews and metaanalyses, can ensure that teaching methods are up to date (Dutra et al., 2022; Koharchik et al., 2014). This includes using the most current research to inform teaching strategies and curriculum design.

The Think-Pair-Share (TPS) strategy involves students thinking about a problem individually, then discussing it with a partner before sharing their findings with the larger group (Alsolais, 2024). This method enhances understanding through collaborative problem solving and peer teaching, which can significantly improve drug dosage calculation skills.

Using simulations and virtual case studies provides a realistic context for practicing drug calculations (Zahara-Such, 2013). This approach helps students apply their knowledge in practical scenarios, improving their ability to perform accurate calculations in clinical settings.

Low-fidelity simulations, such as paper-based or computer-based exercises, offer a cost-effective way to practice drug calculations. These simulations can be used to provide repeated practice opportunities, which are essential for mastery of the skill. Role play exercises where students can practice communication and decision-making skills in a safe environment can also be beneficial, allowing them to develop interpersonal skills related to medication administration and accurate calculations.

SCENARIO-BASED LEARNING

Scenario-based learning is an effective pedagogical approach that can significantly reinforce drug calculation skills in nursing students by providing a realistic and contextually relevant learning experience. This type of learning offers immersive and realistic contexts by utilising high-fidelity virtual simulations that replicate real clinical environments. These simulations can present various patient scenarios requiring accurate drug calculations, such as administering IV medication, calculating dosages for paediatric patients, or managing complex medication regimes. Case studies can be incorporated that require students to apply their drug calculation skills in a clinical context, including consideration of patient histories, laboratory results, and specific medication orders that students must then accurately interpret and act upon.

These scenarios provide hands-on practice opportunities in a controlled environment, which can include mannequins or simulation software to practice medication administration and dosage calculations. The practical application of knowledge helps solidify theoretical understanding. Scenarios also offer immediate feedback on students' calculations and actions within the simulation. This allows students to correct mistakes in real time and understand the consequences of their decision, thereby improving their accuracy and confidence.

Scenarios can be designed involving more complex drug calculations that require critical thinking. For example, scenarios could involve multiple medications with different dosing schedules or patients with multiple comorbidities that affect drug metabolism. This encourages students to make informed decisions based on their knowledge and drug calculations. It helps them develop the ability to prioritise tasks and manage time effectively in high-pressure clinical settings.

Collaborative learning can take place by utilising simulation by bringing groups of students together to solve drug calculation problems, promoting peer learning, and allowing students to learn from each other's approaches and strategies. By conducting debriefing sessions after simulation to discuss what went well and what could be improved, this also aids reflective practice, reinforcing learning and addressing misconceptions.

By ensuring that the scenarios link directly to practice, it provides the connection between theory and practice, showing clearly that what is taught in the classroom can be taken to practice. This helps students see the practical application of their studies and understand the importance of accurate drug calculations in patient care. Scenarios can also support continuous learning by reinforcing previously learned concepts and introducing new ones.

This teaching method provides a safe and supportive environment where students can practice without fear of real-world consequences, helping reduce maths anxiety and build confidence in their ability to perform accurate drug calculations. The use of positive reinforcement encourages students by highlighting their success, motivating them to continue practicing and improving their skills.

Although scenario-based learning is a powerful teaching method, it does have several limitations when used to teach or reinforce drug calculations.

Complex scenarios can be overwhelming, especially for students who are still developing their foundational maths skills. This can lead to cognitive overload, making it difficult for students to focus on the calculations themselves. Scenarios can often include a lot of information that can distract students from the care task of performing accurate drug calculations. Targeting the difficulty level can be challenging, as students enter nursing programmes with varying levels of maths proficiency and scenarios that are too easy or too difficult for certain students may not be effective in improving their existing skills.

If proper guidance is not provided for the simulation exercise, students may not fully understand the key concepts and steps involved in drug calculations, which can lead to confusion and errors in those calculations. There is a need for skilled facilitators to guide students through scenarios and provide timely feedback to avoid diminishing the learning outcomes.

Developing and implementing high-quality scenarios requires significant time and resources, which can be challenging for educational institutions with limited resources. Scenarios can also be time-consuming to complete, which can add feasibility issues for larger groups of students and the constraints of a typical nursing curriculum that is already densely populated. Some students may require more time to process and understand the scenarios while others may grasp the concept quickly, which can create disparities in learning outcomes and affect the time it takes to undertake the activity.

Whilst scenarios aim to mimic real clinical settings, they may not fully capture the complexity and unpredictability of actual clinical situations. This can limit the transferability of skills learned in scenarios to real-world practice. Scenarios may not fully replicate the emotional and psychological pressures that nurses face in real clinical settings, which can affect their performance in simulated drug calculations and real practice.

TECHNOLOGY-ENHANCED LEARNING

TEL encompasses a wide range of digital approaches, such as e-learning modules, virtual simulations, and online assessments (Kirkwood & Price, 2014). Freeman (2025) conducted a study focusing on immersive TEL delivered through 360-degree video, accessed via both desktop computers and virtual reality headsets, allowing students to observe medication calculations and administration as they unfold in authentic clinical environments. These digital experiences enable repeated exposure to complex, realistic scenarios without compromising patient safety, supporting a pedagogical model grounded in cognitive rehearsal and situated awareness (Freeman, 2025).

Freeman (2025) found that although there were variable improvements in medication accuracy following the delivery of the learning, with immersive TEL demonstrating promise in enhancing realism and engagement in clinical numeracy education, its effectiveness depended on more than delivery format. Freeman (2025) advised that to be truly impactful, TEL must be embedded within a broader pedagogical framework that values inclusion, reflection, feedback, and identity formation, and that educational technologies cannot replace good teaching, but when used thoughtfully, they can extend its reach and relevance.

The following link can be used to access the preceding resources developed by Sean Freeman, requiring an NHS email address to register:

PEARLS

https://tinyurl.com/UoGMMedicine

Teaching Resources to Support Knowledge and Understanding

To reinforce learning, practice problems and quizzes covering topics where teaching has been delivered can help provide opportunities for students to apply what they have learned and see their ability developing.

Interactive content in the classroom, and accessible away from the classroom, helps students engage with the content and practice their skills in a more dynamic way. This might include online tasks, access to worksheets, or scenario-based problems to which students can apply their knowledge and understanding.

Video tutorials can be used to demonstrate how to perform specific calculations or solve common nursing maths problems, and can be helpful because they can be utilised by students as many times as needed and revisited for revision purposes. Such tutorials also offer a more visual learning experience for those students who find this an easier way to learn, providing step-by-step visual guidance to the processes involved in the calculations.

Using real-world examples and authentic and realistic scenarios that nurses commonly encounter in practice can help students see the relevance of the maths skills they are learning and show that the skills are useful to them. Simulation and online virtual learning platforms are ideal for these real-world scenarios to play out in a safe space and provide remote and virtual learning opportunities.

Resources lists for students can provide further support and additional practice for students who need it. Library resources such as textbook lists that explain processes and often include examples and practice questions will support some learners to build their confidence in undertaking a skill they might find particularly difficult. Links to online resources can also be helpful, as many provide built-in practice opportunities as supplementary learning material.

Assessment Strategies

Educators can employ a variety of strategies to assess and improve the mathematical skills of student nurses, especially those with varying levels of maths ability.

Administering pretests at the beginning of a course or module can help identify the initial skill levels of students. Posttests can then be used to measure improvements and identify areas that still need attention and improvement.

Regular quizzes and activities to do outside of the classroom environment, alongside in-class activities, can provide ongoing feedback to both students and the educator about student progress, understanding, and development. Any areas identified as requiring improvement can then be addressed through new activities or guidance to existing activities. Mobile apps can provide on-the-go practice and assessment opportunities, and can include features such as flashcards, practice problems, and real-time feedback.

Encouraging students to reflect on their own learning and assess their own understanding can help them have an awareness of their own strengths and weaknesses. Ideas to support this include reflective journals or diaries, or self-assessment quizzes. Encouraging the use of digital portfolios where students can document their learning process, including their mathematical problem-solving activities, can provide a comprehensive view of their progress and areas needing improvement.

Peer learning is an invaluable tool for increasing knowledge and understanding of maths skills. This collaboration and peer review approach to problem solving can help students learn from each other and gain different perspectives on solving mathematical problems that educators may not be confident in exploring or explaining.

PEER LEARNING

When students teach each other, they often gain a deeper understanding of the material themselves. Explaining concepts to peers can reinforce their own knowledge and highlight areas where they may need further study. However, problems can arise when peers are not well versed in the material. In such cases, they may inadvertently spread incorrect information, which can lead to the reinforcement of misconceptions and errors in drug calculation.

Peer learning encourages collaborative problem solving, which can lead to the development of different strategies for solving drug calculation problems. This can help students see multiple approaches to the same problem, enhancing their problem-solving skills. However, students have varying levels of proficiency in drug calculation skills, and peer learning may not be equally beneficial for all participants. Those who are less proficient may not receive the necessary support to improve.

Learning in a peer group can reduce the anxiety associated with mastering complex drug calculation skills. Peer support can provide a safe environment for asking questions and making mistakes, which can boost confidence in ability. Peer learning does, however, lack the structured guidance and oversight provided by educators, and without proper facilitation, peer learning sessions may become unproductive or off topic.

Peers can also provide immediate feedback and help correct misunderstanding or errors in real time, which can be particularly beneficial for drug calculations, where accuracy is crucial. The effectiveness of this approach relies heavily on the competence and reliability of the peers involved; if the peer group lacks strong leadership or expertise, the learning experience may be less effective.

Engaging in peer learning helps students develop their communication and interpersonal skills, which are essential for effective teamwork in clinical settings.

Group dynamics can sometimes lead to conflicts or uneven participation, where some students may dominate the discussion while others remain passive. This can hinder the learning experience for all participants.

Improvement Strategies

Tailoring teaching methods to the diverse needs of students can help address varying levels of proficiency. This might include providing additional support for those who struggle and more challenging material to those who excel, introducing differentiated instruction to be fully inclusive of everyone's skill level.

Using interactive tools such as online simulations, virtual laboratory environments, and interactive whiteboards can make learning more engaging and help students visualise mathematical concepts rather than relying on verbal description.

Implementing strategies to reduce maths anxiety, such as positive reinforcement, creating a supportive learning environment, and providing reassurance, can help students have more confidence in their abilities and overcome anxiety.

Introducing educational technology such as maths apps, online tutorials, and education software can provide additional resources and practice opportunities for students.

Providing timely and constructive feedback on assessments and practice papers can help students understand their mistakes and learn from them. This can be done in various ways, such as through one-on-one meetings, written comments, and digital feedback tools, or involving students in the marking process of practice papers, either their own or swapping with peers.

As an educator, it is prudent to confirm that your own knowledge and understanding is up to date both in teaching maths skills and in pedagogical strategies, which helps ensure that students are receiving the best-quality teaching and instruction and that support is appropriate.

Using AI

AI can assist student nurses in becoming proficient in drug calculations in a variety of ways and is not something that educators or students should be afraid of using to support learning both in and out of the classroom.

AI can provide interactive modules that allow students to practice drug calculations in a safe environment with the benefit of providing instant feedback and explanations for any incorrect answers provided. A student can simply ask AI to create questions. For example, typing in "Please provide me with drug calculation questions to calculate the number of tablets that need to be given" will result in a question set that students can then complete. For verification purposes the student simply needs to ask AI for the answers (e.g., "Please can you give me the answers to these?"), and the AI tool will not only provide the correct answers but also explain how the correct answer is calculated, providing students with unlimited practice opportunities.

By taking advantage of these AI capabilities, student nurses can enhance their understanding and proficiency in drug calculations, ultimately improving their confidence and competence in clinical settings.

AI FOR MORE COMPLEX FORMULAS AND ALGORITHMS

AI-powered tutoring systems can play a significant role in helping student nurses master complex drug calculation formulas and algorithms, as such systems can assess a student's current knowledge and adapt the curriculum to focus on areas where they struggle. This personalised approach ensures that students receive targeted practice on complex formulas and algorithms.

AI tutoring systems offer support with more complex formulas by being able to break them down into manageable steps, guiding students through each part of the process. This helps reinforce understanding and builds confidence in students' ability to tackle difficult problems.

Students can receive immediate feedback on their calculations, allowing them to learn from mistakes in real time. This instant correction helps solidify their understanding of the correct methods and formulas rather than waiting for the availability of an in-person tutor or peer support and remembering processes and calculations.

AI systems can generate a wide variety of practice problems, including real-world scenarios that require the application of complex drug calculations. This variety helps students become familiar with different contexts in which these calculations are used. AI can also incorporate visual aids, such as graphs and charts, to help students visualise complex concepts. Simulations can also provide a practical context for applying drug calculations in clinical settings.

AI systems can curate and recommend additional resources, such as videos, articles, and interactive modules, that align with the student's learning needs and preferences and can be available anytime and anywhere, providing students with the flexibility to learn at their own pace and convenience.

By incorporating game-like elements, AI can make learning more engaging. Challenges, rewards, and competitive elements can motivate students to practice more frequently and persistently.

Integrating gamification into simulated learning environments enriches and diversifies learning opportunities for students (Freeman et al., 2024). Freeman et al. (2024) produced a series of game-based resources and evaluated the experiences of them on student learning, finding that the approach improved knowledge and confidence in applying procedures in practice. The games were based on an escape room concept whereby students had to accurately navigate the scenario to escape, with participants reporting improvements in cognitive processes, as well as communication skills, and feeling more prepared for real-life experiences as a result (Freeman et al., 2024).

Effective Online Resources

Next, a selection of links and descriptions to online resources that can support students is presented. You may be aware of others, as this is not an exhaustive list.

Khan Academy offers comprehensive tutorials and practice exercises on a wide range of mathematical topics including arithmetic, algebra, and geometry. This site is useful for foundational maths skills and dosage calculations.

PEARLS

https://www.khanacademy.org

BBC GCSE Bitesize provides interactive lessons and practice questions on basic maths skills that are essential for nursing students. The site covers topics such as fractions, decimals, percentages, and ratios.

PEARLS

https://www.bbc.co.uk/bitesize

Some websites offer specific practice problems related to nursing calculations, including dosage calculations, IV flow rates, and conversions between units and measurement systems:

PEARLS

https://drugcalcsnurses.co.uk
https://london.hee.nhs.uk/sites/default/files/practice_drug_calculations_0.pdf
https://www.registerednursern.com/dosage-calculations-nursing-comprehensive-quiz/
https://testandcalc.com/quiz/testmet.htm
https://www.mathcentre.ac.uk/students/courses/health/drugdose/
https://study.sagepub.com/starkingskrause4e/student-resources/chapter-questions

WolframAlpha is a computational knowledge engine that can help students solve complex maths problems and understand the various steps of calculation. This engine is useful for more advanced mathematical concepts.

PEARLS

https://www.wolframalpha.com

YouTube has channels dedicated to nursing maths, such as "Dosage Calculations Nursing", providing video tutorials that explain mathematical concepts and problem-solving techniques concisely.

PEARLS

https://www.youtube.com/playlist?list=PLQrdx7rRsKfUYdl0TZQ0Tc2-hLIXlHNXq

Mathway is an online tool that provides step-by-step solutions to maths problems, which can be quite helpful for students who need to understand the processes of solving particular types of problems.

PEARLS

https://www.mathway.com/BasicMath

Photomath is available as an app that allows students to scan problems in and receive step-by-step explanations to help break down the problems and allows learning on the go.

PEARLS

https://photomath.com

DosageHelp.com provides a dosage calculations tutorial, complete with explanations and examples, to help nursing students prepare for a medication exam. The site includes topics such as unit conversions, IV infusions, weight dosages, and practice questions.

PEARLS

https://www.dosagehelp.com

Lincoln Memorial University has an online resource of a 39-page practice worksheet from the nursing programme that includes answers to the problems at the end of the worksheet.

PEARLS

https://www.lmunet.edu/caylor-school-of-nursing/documents/Dosage_Calculations_Packet.pdf

ProProfs IV Drip Rate Calculation Practice Quiz is designed for nursing students, healthcare professionals, or anyone interested in improving their skills in drip rate calculations and IV fluid management. It is a practice quiz aimed at reinforcing understanding and application of IV calculations, ensuring that participants are well prepared for real-world scenarios in medical settings.

PEARLS

https://www.proprofs.com/quiz-school/story.php?title=iv-drip-rate-calculations-ttck-pnp

Nurseslabs IV Flow Rate Calculation Reviewer and Quiz includes practice questions for IV flow rate calculations and formulas, aiming to help student nurses review and test their competence. The nursing test bank is separated into two quizzes with 30 questions each.

PEARLS

https://nurseslabs.com/iv-flow-rate-nclex-practice-quiz/

Nurseslabs also has a drug dosage calculations quizzes page, which has practice dosage calculation problems to measure competence in nursing maths.

PEARLS

https://nurseslabs.com/drug-dosage-calculations-practice-quiz/

Online resources aimed at providing supportive information, knowledge, and skill development in relation to basic maths are often aimed at a younger audience and can be inappropriate for adult learners. For students who already feel anxious, are struggling, and may believe that they should already have this knowledge, these types of online resources are not always helpful, so careful selection is wise to avoid escalating any feelings of inadequacy.

Interactive Resources

The next selection of links and suggestions includes sites or ideas that offer a more interactive element to them.

DOSAGE CALCULATION COMPETENCY TEST MODELS

Models such as those presented by Jarvis et al. (2021) can be used as online resources that are self-directed, helping students improve their dosage calculations skills through practice tests and immediate feedback. The models are designed to enhance mathematical competency and confidence in nursing students.

NURSING SCHOOL GAME NIGHT WITH PRIZES

The Dosage Calculation Workshop: NCLEX Game Night is an interactive offering involving dosage calculation challenges and can be played using two devices (ideally a laptop to see the questions and a phone or tablet to enter answers using Kahoot!). This offering makes learning maths skills more engaging by incorporating a competitive and rewarding element. The game night ran live, but educators can create their own versions using the link to see the original version:

PEARLS

https://www.youtube.com/watch?v=_tFAbSPglUI

REGISTEREDNURSERN.COM WITH NURSE SARAH

The Registered Nurse RN website includes videos for solving dosage and calculation problems, along with individual worksheets for each of the videos. The worksheets are in pdf format and have a link to the relevant video, including topics such as unit conversions, dosage calculations, and IV infusions, with nine videos and worksheets in total.

PEARLS

https://www.registerednursern.com/worksheets

SOUTHWEST TECH MATH/SCIENCE RESOURCES

Southwest Wisconsin Technical College offers a teaching and learning resource with drug calculations worksheets that can be used for additional practice. Each worksheet comes with a separate answer key, and some also feature companion videos.

PEARLS

https://swtcmathscience.wixsite.com/swtcmath/drug-calculation-worksheets-videos

Benefits to Students

Using online resources to supplement and support teaching and learning offers several benefits for nursing students to improve their maths skills.

Online platforms often provide personalised learning experiences, allowing students to work at their own pace and focus on areas where they need the most improvement. This individualised approach can help build confidence and proficiency in mathematical skills.

Online platforms offer instant feedback on practice problems, which helps students understand their mistakes and learn from them immediately. This is particularly beneficial for mastering dosage calculations and other critical maths skills in nursing, allowing repeated practice with feedback each time.

These platforms often use more interactive and engaging content than can be delivered in a classroom, such as gamification and simulations, making learning more interesting and enjoyable.

Online platforms can be accessed anytime and anywhere, giving the advantage of making it easier for students to fit maths practice into their already busy schedules. This is paramount to those students who have other commitments or study remotely.

Many platforms offer data analytics to track student progress and provide insights into areas that need improvement. This can help both students and educators identify specific skills that require more attention and tailor future instruction according to that need.

Online platforms also often offer real-world scenarios and case studies that simulate the types of maths problems nursing students will encounter in clinical settings. This helps students develop their critical thinking and problem-solving skills needed for safe and effective medication administration.

By providing a supportive and nonjudgemental learning environment, these tools can help reduce maths anxiety, which is a common issue in nursing students, leading to improved performance and confidence in their mathematical abilities.

Limitations to Students

Although there are many benefits to online resources that students can access away from the classroom, there are some drawbacks or limitations to these resources.

Technical issues to consider include students facing challenges relating to inadequate access to technology or unreliable internet connectivity, which can disrupt the learning process and lead to frustration and disengagement from future activity. Some students may also lack the necessary computer skills to effectively use online platforms, which can hinder their ability to engage with the material.

The absence of face-to-face interaction with peers and educators can lead to feelings of isolation and diminish the sense of community and support that is often found in traditional education settings, such as classroom environments. Alongside this barrier, online platforms often lack the ability for educators to monitor progress and knowledge, which can make it difficult for educators to gauge students' understanding and provide appropriate support.

Accessing these additional online resources requires strong self-discipline from students and good time management skills. Many students already find it challenging to balance their studies with other responsibilities, leading to poor academic performance and increased stress, and the need to access additional resources may only add to their stress. This is particularly relevant when we consider nursing students, as they often are more mature students with family responsibilities.

The home environment can be filled with distractions that can impede focused learning for students, which may result in students finding it difficult to maintain concentration and productivity when accessing resources.

Mitigation Strategies

An awareness of the preceding limitations allows mitigating strategies to be implemented to help students overcome these barriers and manage their learning effectively.

Institutions can offer technical support through IT departments for additional learning platforms added to access resources. They can also offer support with connectivity and device issues. Materials can be provided in an alternative format to support those with limited access to the internet, which can be beneficial. Resources can be obtained by educators and made available on platforms already accessed by students in a format that could be printed on campus facilities, negating the need for internet access at home to complete.

Training and guidance can be provided in the classroom environment by educators to direct students to the resources, demonstrating how to access and utilise the key resources, thus addressing the issues of poor computer literacy.

Creating opportunities for social interaction through virtual study groups and online discussion boards can generate a community feel for the resources, where they can be discussed and peer support can be provided for access issues.

Providing students with time management tools and resources, such as planners and scheduling apps, can help them better manage their time and responsibilities, allowing them to create and protect time for accessing resources.

Implementing regular check-ins with students to monitor their progress helps address issues around educators not having an awareness of the resources accessed or their effectiveness. This also provides an opportunity for further guidance to be given to help students stay motivated and on track with their learning.

Classroom discussions around good study techniques can help ensure that students set themselves up at home with a dedicated study space to help minimise distractions and improve focus. A reminder of the need for regular breaks can be included as well, as this will help students maintain their concentration and productivity during study sessions.

Pocket Guide to Drug Calculations

Discussed in Chapter 7 was a pocket guide to drug calculations, which I created as a physical resource to support students who find asking for help particularly challenging. That chapter detailed the feedback and usefulness of the pocket guide, but here the details of the resource are outlined:

- The resource is credit card size when folded (Fig. 8.1) but opens to a size similar to A4 paper with three sections on each side.
- One side shows unit conversions, tablets/capsules, and weight-based calculations (Fig. 8.2).
- The other side shows the volume to give, flow rates, and drop rates (Fig. 8.3).

The pocket guide provides quick and easy access to essential formulas, conversion charts, and step-by-step instructions for drug calculations. The guide is particularly

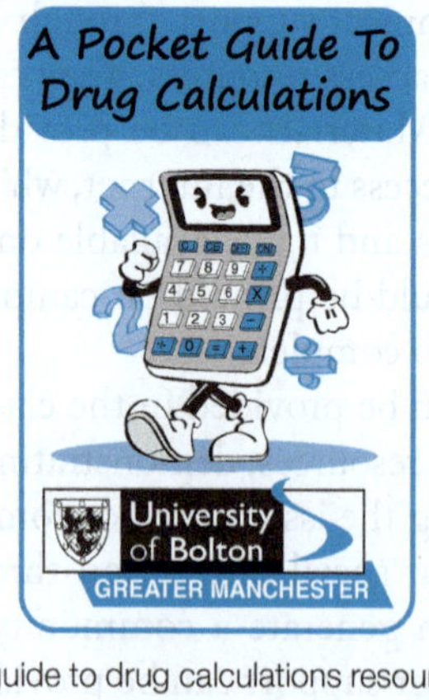

Fig. 8.1 Outside cover of the pocket guide to drug calculations resource. (With permission from University of Bolton, Greater Manchester.)

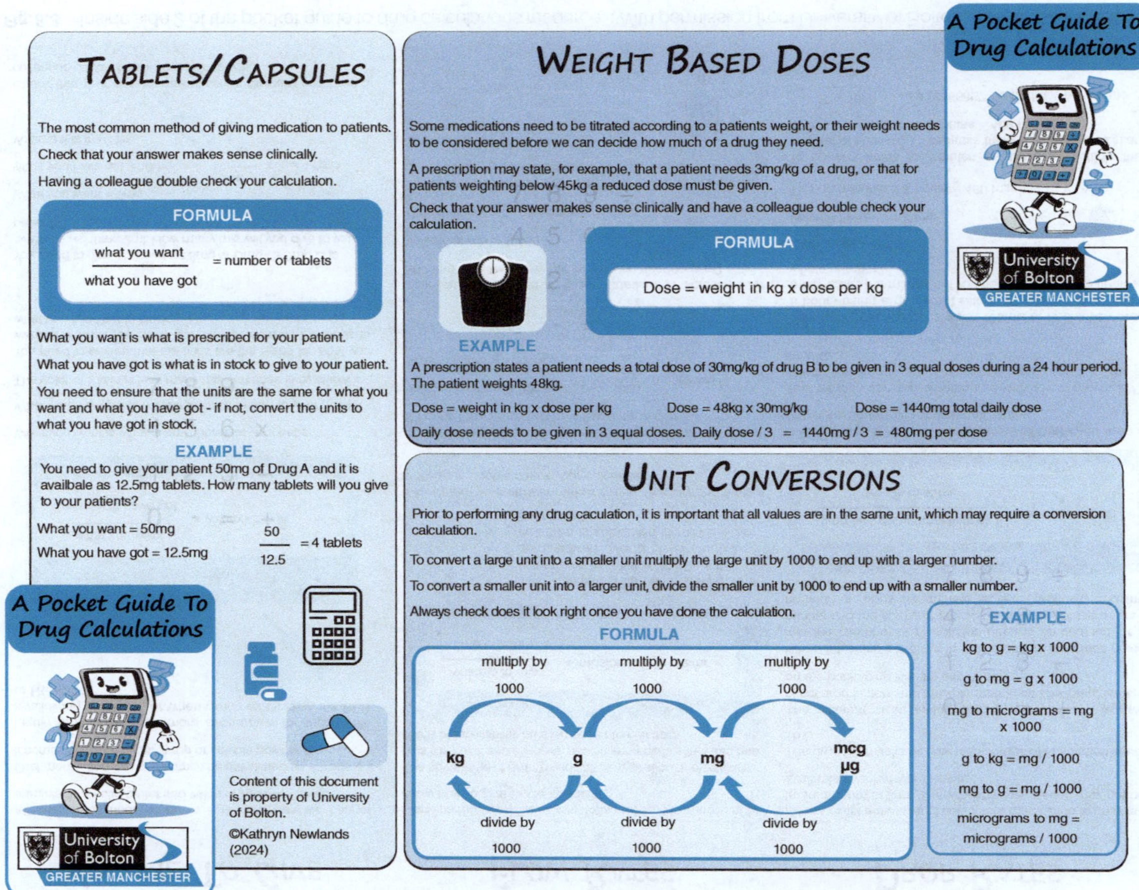

Fig. 8.2 Inside side 1 of the pocket guide to drug calculations resource. (With permission from University of Bolton, Greater Manchester.)

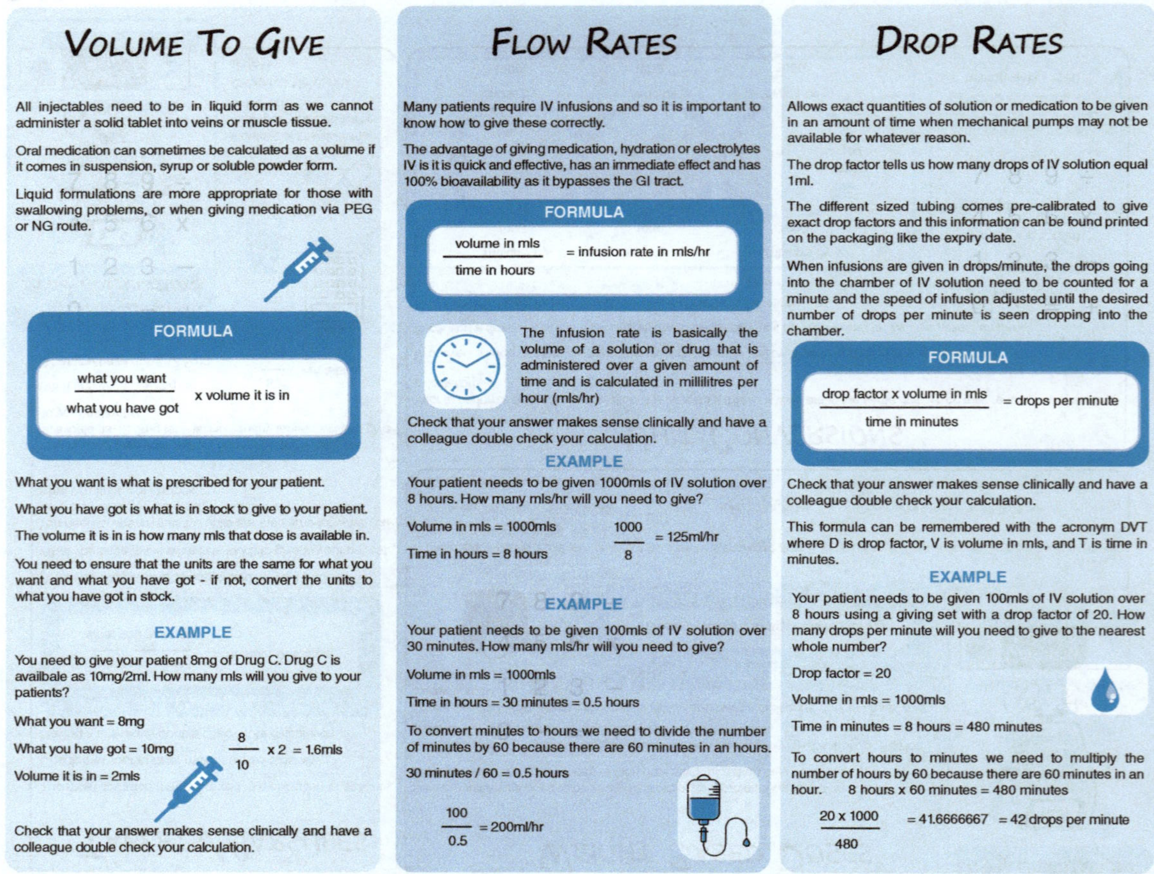

Volume To Give

All injectables need to be in liquid form as we cannot administer a solid tablet into veins or muscle tissue.

Oral medication can sometimes be calculated as a volume if it comes in suspension, syrup or soluble powder form.

Liquid formulations are more appropriate for those with swallowing problems, or when giving medication via PEG or NG route.

FORMULA

$$\frac{\text{what you want}}{\text{what you have got}} \text{ x volume it is in}$$

What you want is what is prescribed for your patient.

What you have got is what is in stock to give to your patient.

The volume it is in is how many mls that dose is available in.

You need to ensure that the units are the same for what you want and what you have got - if not, convert the units to what you have got in stock.

EXAMPLE

You need to give your patient 8mg of Drug C. Drug C is availbale as 10mg/2ml. How many mls will you give to your patients?

What you want = 8mg

What you have got = 10mg

Volume it is in = 2mls

$$\frac{8}{10} \text{ x 2 = 1.6mls}$$

Check that your answer makes sense clinically and have a colleague double check your calculation.

Flow Rates

Many patients require IV infusions and so it is important to know how to give these correctly.

The advantage of giving medication, hydration or electrolytes IV is it is quick and effective, has an immediate effect and has 100% bioavailability as it bypasses the GI tract.

FORMULA

$$\frac{\text{volume in mls}}{\text{time in hours}} = \text{infusion rate in mls/hr}$$

The infusion rate is basically the volume of a solution or drug that is administered over a given amount of time and is calculated in millilitres per hour (mls/hr)

Check that your answer makes sense clinically and have a colleague double check your calculation.

EXAMPLE

Your patient needs to be given 1000mls of IV solution over 8 hours. How many mls/hr will you need to give?

Volume in mls = 1000mls

Time in hours = 8 hours

$$\frac{1000}{8} = \text{125ml/hr}$$

EXAMPLE

Your patient needs to be given 100mls of IV solution over 30 minutes. How many mls/hr will you need to give?

Volume in mls = 1000mls

Time in hours = 30 minutes = 0.5 hours

To convert minutes to hours we need to divide the number of minutes by 60 because there are 60 minutes in an hours.

30 minutes / 60 = 0.5 hours

$$\frac{100}{0.5} = \text{200ml/hr}$$

Drop Rates

Allows exact quantities of solution or medication to be given in an amount of time when mechanical pumps may not be available for whatever reason.

The drop factor tells us how many drops of IV solution equal 1ml.

The different sized tubing comes pre-calibrated to give exact drop factors and this information can be found printed on the packaging like the expiry date.

When infusions are given in drops/minute, the drops going into the chamber of IV solution need to be counted for a minute and the speed of infusion adjusted until the desired number of drops per minute is seen dropping into the chamber.

FORMULA

$$\frac{\text{drop factor x volume in mls}}{\text{time in minutes}} = \text{drops per minute}$$

Check that your answer makes sense clinically and have a colleague double check your calculation.

This formula can be remembered with the acronym DVT where D is drop factor, V is volume in mls, and T is time in minutes.

EXAMPLE

Your patient needs to be given 100mls of IV solution over 8 hours using a giving set with a drop factor of 20. How many drops per minute will you need to give to the nearest whole number?

Drop factor = 20

Volume in mls = 1000mls

Time in minutes = 8 hours = 480 minutes

To convert hours to minutes we need to multiply the number of hours by 60 because there are 60 minutes in an hour. 8 hours x 60 minutes = 480 minutes

$$\frac{20 \text{ x } 1000}{480} = 41.6666667 = \text{42 drops per minute}$$

Fig. 8.3 Inside side 2 of the pocket guide to drug calculations resource. (With permission from University of Bolton, Greater Manchester.)

useful during clinical practice when students need to make accurate drug calculations quickly and efficiently.

The pocket guide also aims to make calculations more understandable by clearly demonstrating how to complete the calculation, showing the formula and an example to simplify the process. The sections allow students to quickly locate the correct formula for the type of calculation they want to complete.

The examples aim to replicate common calculations undertaken in practice, helping students understand how to apply their knowledge in actual practice, thus enhancing their problem-solving skills. As this is a physical guide, it supports more visual learners who can see the breakdown of the example to apply the steps to their own calculations.

The purpose of the pocket guide is multifunctionality, being compact enough that it can be carried around and utilised in classrooms, in clinical practice, or whilst studying in various environments. In high-pressure clinical settings, having a quick reference guide can be invaluable because students are able to quickly look up formulas or steps without having to rely on memory alone, reducing the risk of errors.

Regular use of the pocket guide can reinforce learning and build confidence in students' ability to perform drug calculations accurately, which is crucial for safe and effective medication administration. Knowing that they have a reliable resource to refer to can help reduce anxiety and stress related to drug calculations, allowing students to focus on other aspects of study or patient care depending on their location.

The pocket guide covers a wide range of topics and is comprehensive, ensuring that students are well prepared for various situations that may arise in clinical practice, providing them with an invaluable and indispensable resource.

Summary

Assessing student proficiency in drug calculation skills requires a comprehensive approach that evaluates both the accuracy and application of skills.

Accuracy of calculations needs to be assessed to ensure that students can accurately calculate dosages (including solid and liquid medications), convert units, and calculate IV flow rates. This needs to be done without errors; in particular, common errors include decimal placement and unit conversions.

Students need to be able to complete calculations in a timely manner, as efficient calculation is essential in a fast-paced clinical environment, and they need to be integrated seamlessly into overall patient care without compromising the quality of care.

A good indicator of student ability is their self-confidence. High confidence usually correlates with better performance and reduced anxiety in clinical settings. Scores from drug calculation assessments provide a quantitative measure of students' actual proficiency, but students should be able to recognise and correct common error patterns to improve their accuracy.

Students should also be able to incorporate feedback from educators, peers, and instructors to improve their skills, including making necessary adjustments and demonstrating their improved performance over time.

Drug calculations are a skill that needs repeated exposure and practice to gain proficiency, so the skill needs to be revisited regularly to maintain proficiency and reduce the risk of errors.

References

Alsolais, A. M. (2024). Effectiveness of the Think-Pair-Share strategy in enhancing drug dosage calculation skills among student nurses in a public university in Saudi Arabia: An experimental study. *Journal of Healthcare Administration, 3*(2), 176–187. https://doi.org/10.33546/joha.3576

Dutra, S. V. O., Kumar, K., & Clochesy, J. M. (2022). Instruction strategies for drug calculation skills: A systematic review of the literature. *Nurse Education Today, 111*, 105299. https://doi.org/10.1016/j.nedt.2022.105299

Freeman, S. (2025). Evaluating technology-enhanced learning in nursing education: A randomised controlled trial comparing VR, desktop, and face-to-face delivery of medication numeracy instruction. (Unpublished master's dissertation). University of Bolton.

Freeman, S., Fletcher, J., Clouston, K., & Higson, A. (2024). Gamifying simulated nursing education: A digital technology approach to enhancing pedagogy and student experience. *British Journal of Nursing, 33*(4), 206–214. https://doi.org/10.12968/bjon.2024.33.4.206

Jarvis, D. H., McCullough, K. D., & McParland, T. R. (2021). Nurse education and mathematical competency: Implementation of an online, self-directed, prerequisite model. *International Journal of Environmental Research and Public Health, 18*(24), 13106. https://doi.org/10.3390/ijerph182413106

Kirkwood, A., & Price, L. (2014). Technology-enhanced learning and teaching in higher education: What is 'enhanced' and how do we know? A critical literature review. *Learning, Media and Technology, 39*(1), 6–36. https://doi.org/10.1080/17439884.2013.770404

Koharchik, L., Hardy, E., King, M., & Garibo, Y. (2014). Evidence-based approach to improve nursing student dosage calculation proficiency. *Teaching and Learning in Nursing, 9*(2), 69–74. https://doi.org/10.1016/j.teln.2013.12.003

Valcourt, M., Smith, D., Petillo, A., & Caufiled, E. (2023). Improving nursing students' confidence with dosage calculation after implantation of a comprehensive teaching strategy. *International Journal of Nursing and Health Care Research, 6*, 1447. https://doi.org/10.29011/2688-9501.101447

Wright, K. (2005). An exploration into the most effective way to teach drug calculation skills to nursing students. *Nurse Education Today, 25*(6), 430–436. https://doi.org/10.1016/j.nedt.2005.04.004

Zahara-Such, R. M. (2013). Improving medication calculations of nursing students through simulation: An integrative review. *Clinical Simulation in Nursing, 9*(9), e379–e383. https://doi.org/10.1016/j.ecns.2012.08.003

CHAPTER 9

Links to Relevant Governmental and International Bodies

Kathryn Newlands

Introduction

Student nurse attrition remains a significant challenge for healthcare education and workforce sustainability. Understanding the role of governmental and international bodies in shaping policy, funding, and support systems is essential for addressing this issue effectively. This chapter explores key organisations that influence nursing education and retention, highlighting their contributions to improving student outcomes and reducing dropout rates.

The chapter begins by examining UK governmental bodies, including the Nursing and Midwifery Council (NMC), Health Education England (HEE), the Department of Health and Social Care (DHSC), NHS England, and Care Quality Commission (CQC). It explains their roles in setting standards, funding education, and ensuring quality in clinical placements. The discussion then moves to professional organisations such as the Royal College of Nursing (RCN) and the Office for Students (OfS), which advocate for student support and educational quality.

Next, the chapter considers international bodies, such as the World Health Organisation (WHO), International Council of Nurses (ICN), European Federation of Nurses Associations (EFN), and others, outlining their global initiatives to improve nursing education and workforce retention. It also addresses policy and funding mechanisms, both in the UK and internationally, that aim to reduce attrition through financial support, mental health initiatives, and workforce planning.

Further sections explore mental health support programmes, strategies for improving nursing education, and the role of key performance indicators (KPIs) in monitoring and evaluating programme effectiveness. The chapter concludes by summarising how these organisations and policies collectively contribute to creating a more supportive and sustainable environment for nursing students.

This final chapter considers some relevant UK governmental and international bodies that focus on student nursing attrition. These organisations provide valuable resources and guidelines that can help address the challenges of student nursing attrition and enhance the skills necessary for effective nursing practice. It also considers how these organisations address the issue of student nursing attrition through policy and funding.

UK Governmental Bodies

UK governmental bodies work collaboratively to address the challenges of student nursing attrition and support the ongoing professional development of nurses in the UK. In the following, an overview is given on how these organisations work, what their main objectives are, and how they support the improvement of student nurse attrition.

NURSING AND MIDWIFERY COUNCIL

The NMC (https://www.nmc.org.uk/about-us/) is the regulatory body for nurses and midwives in the UK. Their primary role is to ensure that these professionals provide safe and effective care to patients. The functions and responsibilities can impact on student retention in several ways.

The NMC sets and maintains standards for nursing and midwifery education, training, and practice, ensuring that all registered nurses and midwives meet the necessary competencies to provide safe care. By ensuring that nursing education programmes are rigorous and relevant, the NMC helps create a strong foundation for student learning, which can enhance student satisfaction and reduce attrition. They develop and publish standards for education, practice, and conduct for nurses and midwives, guiding professionals in their practice and helping to ensure that high-quality care is delivered. The NMC also requires registered nurses and midwives to engage in continuing professional development to maintain their skills and knowledge, ensuring that they stay current with best practices and developments in healthcare. This instills students with the value on lifelong education.

The NMC is responsible for the registration of nurses and midwives in the UK, maintaining a public register of qualified professionals, ensuring that only those who meet the required standards can practice, in line with public protection, motivating students to complete their education, knowing that they are being trained to meet high standards of care.

The NMC approves and accredits nursing and midwifery education programmes in the UK, including evaluating curricula, teaching methods, and assessment processes to ensure that they meet established standards. This role in accreditation ensures that institutions provide high-quality training and programmes that meet NMC standards and are more likely to engage students effectively, leading to higher retention rates.

Fitness to practice concerns and investigations are part of the role of the NMC, including handling complaints and conducting hearings to determine whether a professional is fit to continue practicing. These regulations help maintain high standards among nursing students, ensuring that they are adequately prepared and supported throughout their education, helping to reduce the likelihood of students dropping out due to academic or professional challenges.

HEALTH EDUCATION ENGLAND

HEE (https://www.hee.nhs.uk/our-work) is responsible for ensuring that the healthcare workforce in England is equipped to meet the needs of patients and the public.

Workforce planning is conducted by HEE to assess current and future healthcare workforce needs, involving analysing data to ensure that there are enough trained professionals to meet the demands of the healthcare system. By conducting workforce planning, HEE ensures that nursing programmes are aligned with the demand for nurses in the healthcare system, supporting institutions to manage student intakes effectively, reducing the likelihood of students feeling overwhelmed or unsupported, which can lead to attrition.

HEE oversees the education and training of healthcare professionals, ensuring that training programmes are aligned with the needs of the NHS and the communities they serve. This includes developing and implementing educational standards and curricula. HEE commissions nursing education programmes and allocates funding to ensure that they meet the high standards. Quality education is crucial for student satisfaction and engagement, which can help reduce dropout rates.

By encouraging interprofessional education, fostering collaboration among different healthcare providers, the learning experience of the student is enhanced, making learning more engaging and relevant, which may help retain students.

DEPARTMENT OF HEALTH AND SOCIAL CARE

The DHSC (https://www.gov.uk/government/organisations/department-of-health-and-social-care) oversees and shapes health and social care policy in England. They develop national health and social care policies aimed at improving the health and well-being of the population, including policies related to public health, mental health, social care, and the NHS. They allocate funding to the NHS and other health and social care organisations, ensuring that resources are distributed effectively to meet the needs of the population and improve service delivery.

They oversee regulatory bodies such as CQC and the NMC, ensuring that healthcare providers meet established standards of care and safety.

Research and innovation in health and social care is supported by the DHSC, which funds initiatives that lead to improved patient outcomes and more effective service delivery. This includes collaboration with various stakeholders, such as healthcare providers, professional organisations, and community groups, to develop policies and initiatives that address the needs of the population. Some of this research focuses on nursing education and workforce issues, the data from which can inform targeted interventions to support at-risk students and improve retention.

The DHSC implements public health initiatives aimed at improving health outcomes, preventing disease, and promoting healthy lifestyles, including vaccination programmes, health education campaigns, and strategies to address health inequalities. They promote the integration of health and social care services to provide more coordinated and comprehensive care for individuals, particularly those with complex needs. Ensuring integrated care models can enhance students' learning experiences and make them feel more connected to their future roles, which attracts more students to nursing programmes. Increased interest in the profession can lead to a more engaged student body, potentially reducing attrition.

The DHSC plays a key role in responding to public health emergencies and crises, such as pandemics or health threats, coordinating efforts to protect public health and ensure the continuity of care. In relation to nursing education, this highlights the importance of various nursing roles and increases awareness of the nursing profession, motivating students to persist in their studies, knowing that their future contributions are vital.

NHS ENGLAND

NHS England (https://www.england.nhs.uk/) is a key organisation within the NHS in England, responsible for overseeing and managing the delivery of healthcare services. They provide strategic leadership for the NHS, setting priorities and direction for healthcare services across England, working to ensure that the NHS meets the needs of the population.

NHS England is responsible for commissioning healthcare services, which involves planning, purchasing, and monitoring services to ensure that they are effective and meet the needs of patients. This includes allocating funding to Clinical Commissioning Groups (CCGs) and other healthcare providers. The organisation then monitors and evaluates the quality of healthcare services, ensuring that they meet established standards, working to improve patient safety and the quality of care across the NHS.

Workforce planning is part of the organisation's responsibilities, ensuring that there are enough trained healthcare professionals to meet the needs of the population, including supporting initiatives to recruit, train, and retain staff. This supports nurse education by ensuring that clinical placements are well structured and supporting, which is essential for practical training and can significantly enhance student confidence and satisfaction, thereby reducing attrition.

NHS England implements public health initiatives and promotes the integration of service provision, creating a more collaborative and supportive environment for nursing students, enhancing their learning experiences, and making them feel more connected to their future roles. They also promote patient engagement and involvement in decision-making processes regarding their care.

CARE QUALITY COMMISSION

CQC (https://www.cqc.org.uk/) is the independent regulator of health and social care services in England with the primary role of ensuring that these services provide safe, effective, compassionate, and high-quality care. They monitor compliance with the Health and Social Care Act and associated regulations, ensuring that providers adhere to legal requirements and best practices in delivering care. They engage with patients, service users, and the public to gather feedback about their experiences with health and social care services, helping to inform inspections and regulatory decisions.

After inspection, CQC provide ratings for services based on their performance, helping the public make informed choices about their care and encouraging providers to improve. If a service if found to be inadequate or poses a risk to patient safety, CQC has the authority to take enforcement actions, including issuing warnings, imposing fines, or even closing services that do not meet expected standards.

CQC reports on its findings, including inspection results and trends in care quality. These reports are made available to the public, promoting transparency and accountability in the health and social care sector.

Results of CQC reports have implications for student nurse attrition, as CQC activities and regulations can influence the educational environment and overall experience of nursing students. Students undertake clinical placements in the settings monitored and reported on by CQC, where high-quality placements that meet CQC standards can enhance students' learning experiences, leading to greater satisfaction and lower attrition rates, and those with inadequate ratings may lead to negative experiences, leading to dissatisfaction and an increase in the likelihood of students dropping out.

ROYAL COLLEGE OF NURSING

Although not a governmental body, the RCN (https://www.rcn.org.uk/) is a professional body and trade union for nurses in the UK with a primary role of advocating for the interests of nurses and nursing as a profession. They represent nurses in discussions with government, healthcare organisations, and other stakeholders to influence health policy and improve working conditions, addressing workforce issues such as staffing levels, pay, and working conditions. They foster a sense of community among nurses by providing networking opportunities, forums, and events to help nurses connect, share experiences, and support one another in their professional journeys.

The RCN provides resources and support for the professional development of nurses, including access to continuing education, training programmes, and professional development opportunities to enhance skills and knowledge. They provide guidance on best practices, clinical standards, and ethical issues in nursing, with resources, publications, and tools to help nurses deliver high-quality care.

The RCN engages with the public to raise awareness of nursing issues and the importance of nursing in healthcare, promoting the value of nursing and advocating for the profession's role in improving health outcomes. They collaborate with international organisations to share knowledge, best practices, and experiences, promoting global nursing standards and supporting the development of the nursing profession worldwide.

These efforts from the RCN have implications for student nurse attrition, as their activities and support can significantly influence the educational experience and overall satisfaction of nursing students. They advocate for high standards in nursing education, promoting quality education and ensuring that programmes are well structured and adequately supported, which can enhance satisfaction and reduce attrition.

Opportunities for professional development are available to students as well as registered professionals, helping nursing students feel more competent and confident in their skills, which may encourage them to complete their programmes. Offering guidance on clinical standards and best practices leads to similar positive outcomes for nursing students.

By advocating for better working conditions for nurses, a more positive environment is created for nursing students during clinical placements, which can enhance their educational experience and reduce attrition, whilst also enhancing a sense of belonging and support for students.

The RCN provides support services, including legal advice and counselling which can help nursing students navigate challenges they may face during their studies. Having access to these resources can alleviate stress and improve student retention. They also facilitate a mentorship programme that connects nursing students with experienced professionals who can provide them with guidance, support, and encouragement, helping students overcome challenges and stay committed to their studies.

OFFICE FOR STUDENTS (OFS)

The OfS (https://www.officeforstudents.org.uk/) is the independent regulator of higher education in England, with a primary role of ensuring that students receive a high-quality education and have a positive experience in higher education institutions.

The OfS regulates universities and colleges to ensure that certain standards of quality and accountability are met, including assessing their financial viability, governance, and academic standards. They work to protect students' interests, ensuring that they have access to high-quality education and that their rights are upheld.

Institutions are monitored by the OfS to ensure that they provide a safe and supportive learning environment, assessing the quality of education provision, ensuring that course delivery meets the needs of both students and employers, and setting out expectations for quality and monitoring compliance. They encourage innovation in teaching and learning and the development of new approaches to education that enhance student outcomes.

The OfS promotes access to higher education for underrepresented groups, working to reduce barriers to entry and improving participation rates among diverse populations, including funding initiatives aimed at widening participation. They focus on enhancing the overall student experience, gathering feedback from students and using this information to inform policy and improve educational practices.

The actions of the OfS impact on student attrition by ensuring that high-quality education is provided, enhancing student satisfaction and engagement with positive learning environments and access to a wider population and thereby reducing the likelihood of attrition. The OfS collects and analyses data on student demographics, outcomes, and experiences which can be used to help identify trends and areas for improvement, allowing implementation of targeted interventions to support students identified at greater risk of attrition.

International Bodies

The following international bodies collaborate with national governments and organisations to develop policies and programmes that support nurses' professional development, and consideration is given as to how they address the challenges of nursing attrition globally.

GLOBAL EQUIVALENCY OF THE NMC

The National Council of State Boards of Nursing (NCSBN) in the United States, the Canadian Nurses Association (CNA), which is a national professional association with each province and territory of Canada having its own regulatory body, the Nursing and Midwifery Board of Australia (NMBA), the Nursing Council of New Zealand, the South African Nursing Council (SANC), the Nursing and Midwifery Board of Ireland (NMBI), the Singapore Nursing Board (SNB), and the Indian Nursing Council (INC) all play crucial roles in ensuring the quality and safety of nursing and midwifery practice, similar to the NMC in the UK, by setting standards for education, licensing, and professional conduct.

WORLD HEALTH ORGANISATION

WHO (https://www.who.int/news-room/fact-sheets/detail/nursing-and-midwifery) is a specialised agency of the United Nations responsible for international public health. They provide leadership on global health matters, setting the agenda for health research, policy, and practice, coordinating international responses to health emergencies and public health challenges. They play a critical role in responding to health emergencies such as disease outbreaks, natural disasters, and humanitarian crises, coordinating efforts to provide assistance and resources to affected countries.

Evidence-based guidelines, standards, and recommendations are developed and published by WHO for health practices, including disease prevention, treatment protocols, and health system strengthening. They monitor global trends and statistics, collecting data on health indicators, disease outbreaks, and health system performance, helping to inform policy decisions and public health strategies. Technical assistance is provided to countries in developing and implementing policies and programmes, helping to build capacity in health systems, including workforce development, disease surveillance, and health service delivery.

WHO promotes and conducts research to advance knowledge in public health and healthcare, supporting the development of new vaccines, treatments, and health technologies to address global health challenges. They advocate for health equality and work to reduce disparities among populations, focusing on addressing social determinants of health and ensuring that all individuals have access to essential health services. This includes promoting health education and awareness campaigns to inform the public about health issues, disease prevention, and healthy lifestyles, providing resources and tools to support health promotion efforts worldwide.

WHO's role can significantly impact student nurse attrition through various initiatives and policies that influence the global nursing education landscape and the healthcare environment. They set international standards for nursing education and practice, ensuring that programmes prepare students effectively, which can enhance student satisfaction and reduce attrition. WHO efforts to improve the workforce and ensure that staff are well trained leads to better support systems for students, making them feel more valued and likely to complete their programmes. By striving to improve global health and lead on policy initiatives, WHO brings increased recognition of the nursing profession, motivating students to persist in their studies and attracting more students into the profession.

INTERNATIONAL COUNCIL OF NURSES

ICN (https://www.icn.ch/) is a global federation of national nursing associations and represents millions of nurses worldwide, advocating for the nursing profession and the health of populations at the global level. They work to influence health policy and promote the role of nurses in healthcare systems, providing resources, education, and support for professional development including offering guidelines, best practices, and continuing education opportunities to enhance nursing skills and knowledge.

International standards are developed and promoted by ICN for nursing education, practice, and ethics, ensuring that nurses are well prepared to provide high-quality care. They support research initiatives that contribute to the evidence base for nursing practice, encouraging the use of research to inform policy and improve patient care. They work to ensure that nursing perspectives are included in health policy discussions and facilitate networking and collaboration among nurses and nursing organisations to provide a platform for sharing knowledge, experiences, and best practices.

ICN advocates for ethical nursing practice and the protection of human rights in healthcare, developing ethical guidelines and supporting nurses to address ethical dilemmas in their practice. They participate in global health initiatives and collaborate with other organisations to address pressing health challenges such as infectious diseases, maternal and child health, and noncommunicable diseases, supporting the building of nursing and healthcare systems particularly in low- and middle-income countries.

ICN initiatives and policies directly influence the educational environment for nursing students, addressing factors that contribute to attrition. By advocating for quality education, promoting professional development, fostering community, and supporting ethical practice, ICN helps create a more positive and engaging experience for nursing students, ultimately reducing dropout rates.

EUROPEAN FEDERATION OF NURSES ASSOCIATIONS

The EFN (https://efn.eu/) is a key organisation representing nurses across Europe. They advocate for the interests of nursing and the nursing profession at a European level, working to influence health policies and ensuring that nursing perspectives are included in decision-making processes. They provide a unified voice for European nurses on issues affecting the profession and healthcare systems.

Standards are developed and promoted by the EFN for nursing education, practice, and ethics across Europe, helping to ensure that nurses are well trained and equipped to provide high-quality care. They collaborate with European institutions such as the European Union (EU) and WHO to address health challenges and promote the role of the nurses in healthcare delivery.

By ensuring that nursing programmes are well structured and meet quality benchmarks, the EFN helps enhance student satisfaction and reduce the likelihood of attrition. They enhance retention by providing resources and opportunities for professional development, making students feel more prepared and supported in their studies.

PAN AMERICAN HEALTH ORGANISATION

The Pan American Health Organisation (PAHO; https://www.paho.org/en/topics/nursing-and-midwifery) is a specialised international health agency that serves as the regional office for the Americas of WHO, providing leadership on public health issues in the Americas, and guiding countries in developing and implementing health policies and programmes to improve health outcomes. They offer technical assistance to member countries in various areas, including disease prevention, health promotion, and health system strengthening, helping countries enhance their public health infrastructure and services.

Health data and statistics for the Americas is collected, analysed, and disseminated by PAHO, data which is crucial for understanding health trends; identifying priorities, and informing policy decisions to prevent and control communicable and noncommunicable diseases in the regions; and developing strategies and programmes to address health threats such as outbreaks, chronic diseases, and environmental health issues. They prepare for and respond to health emergencies, such as natural disasters and disease outbreaks, coordinating regional responses and providing support to affected countries.

PAHO collaborates with governments, nongovernmental organisations, academic institutions, and other stakeholders to address health challenges and promote best practices in public health, contributing to the development of policies at regional and national levels.

These policies and initiatives help improve educational frameworks and advocate for the importance of nursing within public health and engaging students in their public health promotions, all of which contribute to improving student engagement, motivating learning, and reducing attrition.

EUROPEAN UNION

The EU (https://health.ec.europa.eu/index_en) is a political and economic union of member states located primarily in Europe, promoting economic cooperation and integration among member states, and facilitating free movement of goods, services, capital, and people, including the establishment of a single market and a customs union.

The EU promotes the harmonisation of nursing education standards across member states though directives and frameworks such as the European Qualifications Framework ensuring that nursing programmes meet consistent quality standards, which can enhance student confidence and reduce attrition. The EU supports student mobility programmes such as Erasmus+, which allows nursing students to study abroad and gain diverse experiences, gaining exposure to different healthcare systems and educational environments which can enhance student engagement and commitment to their studies.

Through programmes like Horizon Europe, the EU funds research and innovation in healthcare, including nursing education. The findings can support and inform best practice in nursing education, helping institutions develop effective strategies to support students and reduce attrition.

They address healthcare workforce issues, including nursing shortages and workforce planning, and by promoting policies that support the recruitment and retention of nurses, the EU helps create a more stable and supportive environment for nursing students.

COMMONWEALTH SECRETARIAT

The Commonwealth Secretariat (https://thecommonwealth.org/our-work/health) is the principal intergovernmental organisation of the Commonwealth of Nations, which is a political association of 56 member states, most of which are former territories of the British Empire. They promote cooperation on various issues including political, economic, and social matters, serving as a platform for dialogue and collaboration.

They support capacity building in health systems, including strengthening nursing education and training programmes, leading to improved educational quality and better-prepared nursing graduates. They advocate for effective health policies that prioritise the role of the nurses in healthcare delivery, thus enhancing the status and support for nursing education, and encourage the sharing of best practices and research findings related to healthcare and nursing.

The Commonwealth Secretariat's efforts to improve nursing education, support mental health, and enhance career opportunities can contribute to reducing attrition rates among student nurses, ultimately leading to a more stable and effective nursing workforce.

INTERNATIONAL ORGANISATION FOR MIGRATION

While primarily focused on migration issues, the International Organisation for Migration (IOM; https://www.iom.int) also addresses the global health workforce, including nursing, in the context of global health, migration, and the provision of healthcare services to migrants and refugees.

They engage in public health initiatives that address the health needs of migrant populations and provide training and resources to healthcare professionals to enhance their ability to care for diverse populations, including cultural competency training to better understand the unique needs of migrants.

This focus on migration and health can influence nursing education and student experiences, and by addressing the needs of diverse populations, providing adequate support, and fostering a sense of purpose, nursing programmes can help reduce attrition rates among student nurses by preparing them for real-world situations and fostering a sense of purpose and commitment.

UNITED NATIONS EDUCATIONAL, SCIENTIFIC AND CULTURAL ORGANISATION

The United Nations Educational, Scientific and Cultural Organisation (UNESCO; https://www.unesco.org/en) is a specialised agency of the United Nations that aims to promote peace, sustainable development, and intercultural dialogue through international cooperation in education, the sciences, and culture.

Their focus on education, health, cultural diversity, and global collaboration supports the nursing profession by promoting quality education, enhancing cultural competency, and advocating for health equity. These efforts ultimately contribute to better health outcomes and the advancement of nursing as a vital component of healthcare systems worldwide.

UNESCO's focus on quality education, cultural competency, lifelong learning, and global health can positively influence the experiences of nursing students. By addressing factors that contribute to attrition, such as lack of support, inadequate training, and feelings of disconnection, these initiatives can help reduce dropout rates and promote a more stable nursing workforce.

Addressing the Issue of Student Nurse Attrition Through Policy and Funding

UK government and international bodies address the issue of student nursing attrition through various policies and funding initiatives aimed at improving recruitment and retention in the nursing profession. What follows is an overview of some of these manifestations, which aim to create a more sustainable and attractive environment for nursing students, ultimately enhancing the nursing workforce and improving patient care outcomes.

UK GOVERNMENTAL POLICIES AND FUNDING

The NHS Learning Support Fund provides additional financial support to eligible nursing students, offering at least £5000 per year to help cover living costs and educational expenses. This funding is crucial, as nursing students often face significant financial burdens due to tuition fees and the requirement to complete extensive clinical hours, which limits their ability to work part time.

The RCN has advocated for a loan forgiveness model for nursing students who commit to working for the NHS for a specified period after graduation. This initiative aims to alleviate the financial pressures that contribute to high attrition rates among nursing students. Research indicates that such a model could encourage nurses to remain in the profession for an additional 7 to 10 years, significantly impacting workforce stability (RCN, 2025a). In Scotland, Wales, and Northern Ireland, nursing students continue to receive bursaries, which have remained unchanged for years. There are ongoing reviews to assess and potentially increase these financial supports to better meet the needs of nursing students in these regions (RCN Students Committee, 2025b).

The UK government has announced increases in tuition fees, also applicable to nursing courses, meaning a cost of £9535 per year. This increase has raised concerns about its potential impact on student recruitment and retention, as higher costs may deter prospective students from entering the nursing field.

The NHS Long Term Workforce Plan aims to address nursing shortages by increasing the number of training places and improving the overall working conditions for nurses. This includes developing advanced practice roles and enhancing the training and development of nurses to make the profession more attractive.

INTERNATIONAL POLICIES AND FUNDING

WHO emphasizes the importance of a well-trained nursing workforce and provides guidelines and frameworks to improve nursing education globally. Their initiatives often include recommendations for funding and policy reforms to enhance nursing education and retention rates.

ICN advocates for policies that support nursing education and workforce sustainability. They promote international collaboration to share best practices and resources aimed at reducing attrition rates among nursing students.

UK MENTAL HEALTH SUPPORT

Government-funded programmes play a crucial role in supporting nursing students' mental health and well-being, which is essential for preventing attrition in the nursing profession.

The NHS Learning Support Fund provides financial assistance to nursing students, alleviating some of the financial stress that can contribute to mental health issues. By reducing financial burdens, students can focus more on their studies and well-being rather than worrying about their finances.

Many universities and colleges offer government-funded mental health services, including counselling and psychological support specifically tailored to nursing students. These services help students manage stress, anxiety, and other mental health challenges that may arise during their training.

Government initiatives often support wellness programmes that include workshops on stress management, resilience training, and self-care strategies. These programmes equip nursing students with tools to cope with the demands of their education and clinical placements.

Funding may be allocated to establish peer support networks where nursing students can connect with each other, share experiences, and provide mutual support. These networks can foster a sense of community and belonging, which is vital to mental health.

Government funding research initiatives focus on understanding the mental health challenges faced by nursing students. This research informs policy and programme development, ensuring that mental health support is evidence-based and effectively addresses the needs of students.

Some government programmes emphasise the integration of mental health education into nursing curricula. By training nursing students to recognise and address mental health issues, they are better prepared to support their own well-being and that of their future patients.

Programmes that promote work–life balance, such as flexible scheduling for clinical placements and academic responsibilities, can help reduce stress and burnout among nursing students. Government support for such initiatives can enhance students' overall well-being.

Government funding may support crisis intervention services that provide immediate assistance to nursing students facing acute mental health challenges. These services are critical in preventing crises that could lead to attrition.

INTERNATIONAL MENTAL HEALTH SUPPORT

Programmes funded by international governments are instrumental in promoting the mental health and well-being of nursing students, a factor that is key to reducing attrition within the nursing profession.

Organisations like WHO implement global health initiatives that emphasize the importance of mental health in healthcare education. These initiatives often include guidance and frameworks that encourage countries to develop mental health support systems for nursing students.

International funding bodies, such as the Global Fund and various UN agencies, provide financial resources to countries to develop mental health programmes. These funds can be used to create support services specifically for nursing students, including counselling, stress management workshops, and peer support networks.

Research on mental health challenges faced by nursing students is often supported by international programmes. This research helps identify effective strategies and best practices for mental health support, which can be shared across countries to improve nursing education and retention.

International programmes may focus on capacity building by training educators and healthcare professionals in mental health support. This training equips faculty and staff at nursing schools with the skills to recognise and address mental health issues among students, fostering a supportive educational environment.

International collaborations, such as those facilitated by ICN, promote the sharing of resources and strategies for supporting nursing students' mental health. These networks allow countries to learn from each other's experiences and implement successful programmes.

Policies that prioritise mental health in nursing education are advocated by international organisations. By influencing national policies, these organisations help ensure that mental health support is integrated into nursing curricula and that adequate resources are allocated for student well-being.

Some international programmes focus on establishing crisis intervention services that can be accessed by nursing students facing acute mental health challenges. These services are essential for providing immediate support and preventing crises that could lead to attrition.

International initiatives often emphasise the importance of work–life balance for nursing students. Programmes that promote flexible learning options and manageable workloads can help reduce stress and burnout, contributing to better mental health outcomes.

Improving Nursing Education Programmes to Reduce Student Attrition Rates

UK governmental and international bodies employ various strategies to assess and improve nursing education programmes aimed at reducing student attrition rates. These strategies include research, policy development, funding initiatives, and the establishment of standards.

UK GOVERNMENTAL BODIES

The NMC collects data on student enrolment, progression, and attrition rates, which is analysed to identify trends and factors contributing to student dropout, allowing for targeted interventions. The NMC sets standards for nursing education programmes, ensuring that they meet specific quality criteria. Regular reviews and inspections of nursing programmes help maintain high educational standards and identify areas for improvement.

HEE conducts workforce planning and research to understand the challenges faced by nursing students, using this information to inform policy and programme improvements.

The OfS monitors the quality of higher education institutions, including nursing programmes, and ensures that they provide adequate support for student success.

Collaborative efforts between governmental bodies and educational institutions lead to the development of curricula that address the needs of students. This includes integrating mental health education, resilience training, and practical skills development to better prepare students for the challenges of nursing.

Governmental bodies advocate for the establishment of robust support services, including academic advising, counselling, and peer support networks. These services are essential for helping students navigate the demands of nursing education and reducing attrition.

INTERNATIONAL BODIES

WHO and ICN develop global standards and guidelines for nursing education. These frameworks help countries assess and improve their nursing programmes, ensuring that they are aligned with best practices.

International organisations conduct research on nursing education and student attrition, sharing findings and best practices across countries. This collaborative approach allows nations to learn from each other and implement effective strategies to reduce attrition.

Capacity building is often a focus of international programmes, whereby training is provided to educators and healthcare professionals in effective teaching methods, mental health support, and student engagement strategies. This training enhances the quality of nursing education and supports student retention.

International bodies advocate for policies that prioritise nursing education and student well-being. By influencing national policies, they help ensure that adequate resources and support systems are in place to address the challenges faced by nursing students.

International organisations often engage in monitoring and evaluation of nursing education programmes to assess their effectiveness. This includes evaluating student outcomes, satisfaction, and retention rates, which then inform ongoing improvements.

Key Performance Indicators

Various KPIs are used to measure the effectiveness of nursing education programmes both within the UK and internationally in reducing student attrition rates, helping to assess the quality of education, student support, and overall programme effectiveness.

Attrition rates are a primary KPI for assessing the effectiveness of nursing education programmes, looking at the percentage of students who withdraw from programmes before completion. A lower attrition rate indicates better student retention and programme effectiveness.

High completion rates suggest that students are receiving adequate support and resources to succeed in their studies. The completion rate KPI looks at the percentage of students who successfully complete their nursing programme within the expected timeframe.

Student satisfaction surveys are a way to gather feedback from students regarding their educational experience, including the quality of teaching, support services, and overall satisfaction. High levels of student satisfaction are often correlated with lower attrition rates, indicating that students feel supported and engaged with their education.

KPI metrics such as average grades, pass rates for assessments, and performance in clinical placements can be used to provide an indication of effective teaching and learning practices, which may contribute to higher retention rates.

The level of student participation in academic advising, counselling, and other support services offered by the educational institution provides an indicator of engagement, with higher engagement often being associated with lower attrition rates, as students who utilise these services are more likely to be successful in their studies.

Employment outcomes also are a useful KPI with regards to success and attrition, as a higher percentage of graduates who secure employment in nursing or related fields following graduation can reflect the quality of the nursing education programme and its alignment with workforce needs, which can impact and influence future student retention.

Evaluations and feedback from healthcare organisations that host nursing students for clinical placements can be useful, as positive feedback from placement providers can indicate that students are well prepared and supported, which may contribute to lower attrition rates.

KPIs aimed at understanding the data on the diversity of the student population and the effectiveness of initiatives aimed at supporting underrepresented groups can help ensure that all students feel included and supported and can help reduce attrition rates, particularly among marginalised groups.

Metrics related to student mental health, such as the availability and utilisation of mental health services, can be crucial to improving attrition, as addressing mental health needs is crucial to student success and effective programmes should demonstrate positive outcomes in this area.

Comparing programme outcomes with international standards and best practices in nursing education is also key, as benchmarking against global standards helps identify areas for improvement and ensures that programmes meet international quality expectations.

Summary

Having an awareness of national and international organisations can be useful when looking to improve student nurse attrition rates, as these links to organisations can provide guidance and policies to support issues within education.

Although not an exhaustive list of resources, a starting point to some of the major influences in global nursing education and how they can address attrition rates of students has been presented.

References

Royal College of Nursing. (2025a). *Nurses would stay in the NHS for up to 10 extra years if their student loans were 'forgiven', major report finds.* Royal College of Nursing. https://www.rcn.org.uk/news-and-events/Press-Releases/nurses-would-stay-in-the-nhs-for-up-to-10-extra-years-if-their-student-loans-were-forgiven

RCN Students Committee. (2025b). *Resolution: Nursing student financial support.* Royal College of Nursing. https://www.rcn.org.uk/congress/congress-events/nursing-student-financial-support-2025

INDEX

Note: Page numbers followed by '*f*' indicate figures, '*t*' indicate tables and '*b*' indicate boxes.

A

B

C

D

E

V

W